With exams passed and qualifications gained, what more does a doctor need to know? All sorts of things, as the success of the first volume of *How To Do It* showed. Now this second volume brings more expert advice to fill the gaps.

HOW TO DO IT

Volume 2

Published by the British Medical Journal
Tavistock Square, London WC1H 9JR

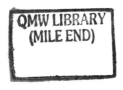
First Edition 1987
Reprinted 1989

ISBN 0 7279 0179 6

Typeset by Eta Services (Typesetters) Ltd, Beccles, Suffolk
Printed in Great Britain by Latimer Trend & Company Ltd, Plymouth

Contents

vii

J E Smeathers, PHD, *research fellow, rheumatism research unit, University of Leeds LS2 9PJ*
D T Thompson, PHD, *training consultant, Stony Stratford MK11 1BQ*

Organise your time

DOUGLAS BLACK

It is lucky for writers of didactic articles, and perhaps also for doctors in general, that we are not rigidly constrained to practise what we preach. For this particular subject I have the uneasy feeling that I must have wasted a good deal of that precious and limited commodity, in excess of what I have been successful in organising. But there are two pleas to be made in mitigation: the possessive pronoun in the title is "your" and not "my"; and I have had the salutary experience of working for and with people who by any standards would be considered to have used their time wisely. So let me try to tell you what I have learnt from them while still making no claim to have emulated them.

A time for every purpose

Perhaps the first thing to recognise is that the greater part of time for most of us is not open to be organised. We are not of course any longer constrained by the old agricultural adage, "Eight hours to work, eight hours to play, eight hours to sleep"—and still less by its tailpiece, "and eight bob a day." But all of us need some sleep, whatever the variation in requirement between individuals. And the balance of opinion is certainly in favour of some equivalent of "play," not discounting, however, those fortunate enough to find their recreation in their work. "Dulce est desipere in loco"*
—and I remember from some years back how a rather tedious faculty discussion on what could be permitted, or not permitted, in an elective period was brought to life by the suggestion from our enlightened dean, Colin Campbell, that provision ought to be left

---

*For, when the time and place are right
  'Tis sweet to make good cheer.—HORACE (Translated by Lord Dunsany.)

for a young man who just wanted to lie in a grassy field and think. But even if we stick to that part of time designated as "work," for most people in most occupations it tends to be organised for them rather than by them. We doctors are more fortunate than most; but it is the rare freelance among us who is not to some extent the creature of the system, and not its creator.

I hope that in saying this I am recognising a fact of life, and not disparaging routine, which is something that we all need. Indeed, it can be wonderfully comforting during the periods when some apparently more creative activity seems to be going badly; I recall how in the days when I did research and things were going badly it was a considerable solace to undertake either a teaching session or an outpatient clinic. But such activities, however comforting and in their own way challenging, are normally dictated by timetable and not by personal initiative and organisation.

Even after making all these deductions for sleep, recreation, and routine, there still remains for most of us some time that we think we can organise. Before I turn to specific aspects of organising time for particular tasks, there is one piece of general advice which could be summarised thus, "Discover your own tempo and work with the grain of it and not against it." I have already mentioned that we need differing amounts of sleep; and it is better to be awake during an examination than to have spent a wakeful night before it in what may be a panic effort at catching up. But we also seem to need sleep at different times of the 24 hour cycle. We may not discover this in the set routine of our schooldays, but in the comparative freedom of the university we soon discover whether we are larks or owls. It is sensible to recognise which we are, and to concentrate as far as possible our most original tasks in our best time of the day. I learnt from Leslie Witts that this is not the same thing as being idle when not at one's best; he was fond of quoting from Matthew Arnold, "... tasks in hours of insight will'd/Can be through hours of gloom fulfill'd."

Another general principle is perhaps to try to devote as much as possible of your disposable time to things that you are good at. The difficulty here, of course, is to discover what these things are. The hedonist in me says, "If you are enjoying doing something, you may be doing it well"; but the puritan in me says, "That may be a necessary criterion, but it's not a sufficient one—you may be enjoying it, and still doing it jolly badly." Self assessment also has the weakness of wishful thinking—I have known superb clinicians who misdiagnosed themselves as researchers, and conversely. It is not always easy for a young man to recognise the direction of his own talents, and it may be the duty of a tutor or the head of a department to help here, difficult though advice of this kind may be to give or to take. Of course with the passage of time more objective evidence may appear—clinical success brings patients, academic success increases the ratio of accepted to rejected papers and communications to societies. I am not, I hope, suggesting that we should attempt only those doors which yield at a touch; but if repeated attempts suggest that they may be locked it might be an idea to try something else. And of course, on a longer time scale, the things which you are good or bad at as a young man may not stay that way thoughout life—even quite foolish people may learn from the rigours of experience.

Academic questions

Coming to more specific matters, as an academic I had to apportion my time among clinical work, research, teaching, and administration. As the more inescapable components, clinical work and teaching run fairly constantly through an academic career; but as time goes on it takes more resolution than I possess to prevent administration from encroaching on the time available for research. For many of us, election to a chair marks the transition from personal to vicarious research, as was crystallised by George Pickering when he told me, "Your job now is to enable other people to do research." Sadly, this must be a task of increasing difficulty for today's professors but it remains a very important part of their responsibility. Discussing their research projects with younger colleagues, and helping them to present their results, is a first call on the time of a professor. Organising time for personal research is very much an individual matter—for some it is an all embracing priority, for others it fluctuates with other interests, and also, let us face it, with how well the research is going. And again, teaching is largely a matter of timetabling and opportunity, not greatly susceptible to personal organisation. May I then devote the rest of this essay to some aspects of the organisation of time spent in clinical work and in administration.

Patients included

The times of ward rounds and of outpatient sessions are usually part of an established hospital framework but the way in which the time so allotted is spent leaves much to individual initiative. What I know of the essentials of clinical organisation I owe to the experience of working for over 20 years with Robert Platt, who taught me that everything must be centred on the patient at the bedside, technical discussion of the illness being reserved for the second half of the round, perhaps over tea. Similarly, in a clinical meeting the worst crime in his eyes was to present a case history without bringing the patient into the conversation.

In the outpatient clinic, working independently, I had of course to make my own discoveries on the use of time—for example, that a teaching clinic, as James Spence emphasised, is an opportunity for one or two students to witness the process of a consultation, not an occasion for giving mini lectures or answering questions on the nature of disease. I learnt that if the day's work is to be done in the day a history must be guided, and not left to free association. More painfully, I occasionally suffered from being at the receiving end of someone else's organisation of their time at my expense—perhaps a cryptic way of describing the situation in which a patient from another hospital staggers into the room laden with 20 pages of notes, a bundle of x rays, numerous investigations on unfamiliar forms—everything but a summary and a statement of the problem. On such an occasion one has to take a deep breath, explain to the patient that there is a lot to look through, apologise for keeping him waiting, and generally do one's best, conscious that the patient is likely to have had his expectations raised by whoever referred him. Managerial and sociological advocates of tight appointments systems, please note.

Boredroom tactics

As in clinical work, so in relation to administration much would seem to be predetermined—the times of boards, committees, examinations, and so on. But individual flexibility creeps in when we consider the way in which the time is actually spent. Because of their critical importance to individuals, I believe that examinations and appointments committees demand the entire concentration of all concerned, and I would be a little worried if an examiner did not feel spent at the end of a day of clinicals and orals. But in most other committees it would be flattering to describe the proceedings as of uniformly high interest. I have never quite had the hardihood to imitate those of my colleagues who visibly get ahead with their correspondence during meetings. I also believe that it is desirable to stay awake, even if arousal is maintained by interest in the people rather than in the business. There is always, too, the possibility that out of a cloudless sky there may come a sudden storm, threatening the body whose interests you are there to represent.

Many years ago I described a syndrome from which I myself suffer—committee insomnia. I have not yet found a cure, but for those who suffer from its opposite (inability to stay awake in committees), I recommend becoming chairman. In that event, however, it is wise to spend a little time beforehand in considering the course that the meeting is likely to take. For major meetings at least, the civil service has a briefing meeting beforehand and a debriefing meeting afterwards; given a competent secretariat, such an array of procedures does more for full employment than for an economical use of collective time.

Seizing the day

Finally, are there ways of "saving time?" Perhaps there are, though it is not easy to prove. Time can certainly be lost by frequent interruptions and by lack of concentration—so you can make use of train journeys and plane journeys and, more riskily, of car journeys along familiar daily routes. Time spent in sleep may not be wasted, even intellectually—nocturnal solutions of a problem have been described. I have sometimes noticed that unusually clear formulations come to mind on first waking—and not all of them are transient, even if they mostly fade into the light of common day.

Take a teaching ward round

JOHN REES

The traditional form of teaching in British medicine has been an apprenticeship and for many specialties the cornerstone of this teaching has been the ward round. This approach of basing teaching on close contact with patients is not typical of medical teaching in all countries, and in some British schools there has been an unfortunate drift away from the bedside and into the lecture theatre and seminar room. Medical educationalists have emphasised the importance of problem based learning—which is the essence of patient based teaching ward rounds where the problem presented by the patient has to be not only dealt with but identified in the first place.

What makes a good ward round? We all have memories from our own student days, many relating to charismatic, sometimes fearsome, consultants' ward rounds but these memories often include the patients and their conditions. Our recall of these patients presented on rounds, far superior to our memory of pages of textbooks, testifies to the effectiveness of those teaching rounds.

The medical curriculum is becoming more and more crowded as everybody wants to teach the essential facts of his specialty. A course covering all possible options would have to be several years longer than at present, and teachers therefore need to be selective and deal with the principles and approaches entailed in different subjects rather than with straight facts. If the division of time in the course is right then during each attachment the student will see on the wards the conditions that are important for hospital practice in that specialty.

There is increasing pressure on teachers' time as well as on students' and you may be tempted to combine business and teaching rounds. Resist this temptation. There is no harm in taking students on business rounds, particularly if they know about all the patients as they should, but don't fool yourself that this can replace their teaching round. It is impossible to devote enough time and thought to teaching in the context of the business round.

There are four main elements to the teaching round; the ward, the patients, the students, and the teachers.

The ward

For many of us cuts in the numbers of beds and shared wards have deprived us of a personal ward and a devoted sister who would control the ward and maintain absolute silence in it during the teaching round. Sanity is best maintained by arranging ward rounds clear of meal times and regular floor polishing sessions. There are advantages in having notes and x ray films available and an accompanying nurse, not least because it introduces the students to a team approach to care.

Hospitals concerned in teaching should have a room available on each ward where the ward round can go to discuss the patients and the problems presented.

Patients

Some patients take great pride in displaying their clinical signs to anyone who shows the slightest interest, but such professional patients are in the minority. Others subject themselves to student ward rounds for a variety of reasons: realisation that students need to learn, obligation to the staff looking after them, and even a worry that refusal may prejudice their future care. Refusal to participate is unusual if patients are consulted beforehand, but they should be given the opportunity to decline. They are more likely to agree if they have a student who sees them regularly and whom they identify as part of the team looking after them.

Patients need to be aware of what is happening in the round. They should be warned that discussion they may hear often applies to general principles and differential diagnoses and not necessarily to their particular case.

Patients to be seen on a ward round are, of course, chosen on the basis of availability. Few patients in hospital are incapable of generating an interesting ward round. There will always be interesting aspects in the history, examination, investigations, social background, or treatment. If not, then there is unlikely to be a good reason for their being in hospital at all.

Some discussion and examination will have to take place at the bedside, but, in general, it is best to move away from the patient to explore the importance of the findings and the management. A side room is best for this, out of earshot of other patients who are less likely to understand the context of a ward round and quite likely to relate a garbled version of the story back to the patient—the ward bush telegraph works at impressive speed and range.

Students

Departments in most hospitals vie with each other to have the largest retinues available for their ward rounds. Anybody in a white coat will do and ability to understand English is not an essential qualification. These large white coated armies have no place on teaching rounds. The optimal number depends a little on the experience of the students but is probably three to five. Larger numbers than this will be unable to see or elicit abnormal physical signs or to take an adequate part in discussion. There is no need for all students to hear a murmur or feel a mass on the round. Once the techniques have been demonstrated and one or two students convinced there is no reason why others cannot return to see the signs for themselves later. Ward rounds should, however, be used to check on the ability of students to elicit histories and to examine.

If learning is really based on patients then students should look after the inpatients on a firm and should be able to present cases without notice. Some units do not run in this way and it is usually best to give prior warning, at least for the main case on the round. This allows the student and the teacher to prepare for the session. Most teachers have some topics that they would prefer not to teach unrehearsed. It is possible to do so but it may limit the directions the round can take.

One of the best stimuli to student learning is the fear of examinations. The ward round has advantages here since it can mimic either short or long case format.

Teachers

The function of the teacher is not to give out information but to inspire the student to do the work. When students have seen and discussed a problem on a ward round they should be left feeling keen to go away and read further on the subject. This sort of patient based or problem based learning sticks much better in the mind because it has some immediacy and interest which reading page by page through a textbook or listening to a formal lecture can never have.

Few medical teachers are taught how to teach and much of their technique comes from their own earlier experience of teachers. There are different approaches but the essential feature is enthusiasm on the part of the teacher. Students will respond to enthusiasm, and learning depends upon the response of the student; it is not a passive transfer of information.

Teaching rounds are not lectures. If you want to give a lecture it is much more comfortable and efficient to move to a lecture theatre and talk to larger numbers. The ward round needs interaction— with the patient, and, most important, with the students. The round can be used to explore points in the history and communication with the patient, to show physical signs, and to explore the techniques of diagnosis and management. Symptoms and signs in a textbook are just components of a list contributing to a diagnosis. In real patients they are individual experiences with their own unique features that can be further explored and interpreted. Few lecturers are gifted enough to bring their descriptions to life in the same way.

The round should be used to explore the students' diagnostic methods and cognitive processes. Students should be taken through the processes they have used to come to their conclusions. As far as possible questions to the students should bring out this exploration, not to force a student's thinking into a rigid format but to let him see the processes he is using and the alternatives available. This form of questioning and exploration is far more valuable than the provision of a list of the causes of clubbing or the familiar "guess what I am thinking of" approach. It is problem based learning and the problem is the patient lying in front of them. Facts and understanding will change during the students' careers, some even before they qualify, but the basic techniques of how to deal with these facts and fit them to patients' needs never change.

The number of patients to be seen on a ward round will vary. A reasonable length for a round is probably about an hour and a half allowing time for hearing the history, demonstrating physical signs, and discussion. This allows time for reasonable discussion of one patient, or two if specific aspects are to be dealt with. Longer rounds are a physical as well as a mental strain.

The great importance of the ward round is that it deals with patients not diseases, it develops thinking processes, and it introduces the approach to patients that most doctors will follow for the rest of their working lives.

Organise a clinical examination

H N COHEN

Chance favours only the mind that is prepared.—PASTEUR

The clinical examination is a trial not only for the candidates but also for the organiser, who has to ensure that candidates receive a fair assessment by providing a careful selection of patients and a calm environment for the examination. He must also ensure that all runs smoothly to allow the examiners to make unbiased judgments on the candidates. The combination of fractious examiners and flustered candidates, as a result of poor organisation, is bound to be detrimental to a candidate's performance.

Three to four months before the examination

Read carefully the examination regulations and any advice given to organisers from the examining body. Efficient organisation requires the cooperation and coordination of several individuals, so once the examination date is known check your own availability and that of your colleagues, nurses, and secretary. You may need to reorganise clinics and holiday and study leave. Try to arrange for the examination to be held in a single ward, used solely for the purpose. Contact the nursing management to arrange for the provision of staff: smooth running on the day greatly depends on an efficient nursing team.

Two to three months before the examination

Prudent organisers will already have a bank of patients to refer to, but, if not, you must start selecting patients at this time. The examining body must tell you the number of candidates and sets of examiners who will be attending; once this is known you must arrange schedules for the patients, who should not have to attend for more than four to five hours, that is, for either a morning or afternoon session. To ask a patient to attend for eight continuous hours is, I believe, reprehensible, and it is unfair to candidates, especially late in the afternoon in "long cases."

Long cases need not have any physical signs, but good histories (and historians) are required. The number of "short cases" per session can be approximately calculated from the following formula:

1.5 × (number of candidates in session + number of sets of examiners).

One long case will generally be needed for each candidate. Any long cases with good physical signs should preferably be used early so that they can be used as short cases later in the session.

Short cases must have clear cut physical signs as it is then easier to test a candidate. Poor candidates show their deficiencies more readily in their inability to recognise clear cut physical signs than in their inability to elicit equivocal abnormalities. At the very minimum, most medical clinical examinations require each candidate to examine cardiovascular, abdominal, neurological, and chest systems.

Once you have decided the days and times that individual patients are required you can send out a letter explaining the examination and suggesting time and date of attendance. Give the patient the opportunity to offer an alternative date in the reply slip and always send a stamped addressed envelope. Make it clear if lunch or transport is to be provided and ask whether these will be required. State the time the patient will be able to leave the examination and never underestimate this.

Keep an up to date list of patients' schedules so that you can reorganise if necessary to ensure a satisfactory number and spread of disease and physical signs. Make sure that the short cases are complete at an early stage. It is an advantage to have some long cases as inpatients at the time of the examination so that a prompt start can be achieved. I always send a second letter to the patients confirming the date and time that they have agreed to come.

Three weeks before the examination

Now comes the arduous task of writing summaries about the patients. These should be concise and consist of relevant information only. Do not use more than one side of A4 paper—and usually considerably less. In short cases one or two lines will suffice, for example, "splenomegaly due to chronic lymphatic leukaemia." There is no need to elaborate; the examiners will assess the patients before the examination starts and make their own notes. The case notes of all long cases and any suitable radiographs or other investigations for long and short cases should be available.

Scripts of case summaries should be stapled together (long cases first), with a contents page at the front listing all patients, their diagnoses, and a number code that corresponds to bed numbers in the ward. There should also be a page showing the ward plan with beds clearly marked with their numbers. Always have a blank top sheet to prevent candidates seeing the contents page.

Check that nurses and porters know about the transfer of patients from ward to ward and the number of patients who will need lunch. If the regulations require it, obtain name badges and white coats for the examiners. Arrange to have well printed, clearly written numbers to put on to beds corresponding to the bed numbers on the ward plan. Earmark side rooms for each pair of examiners and a waiting room for candidates. Arrange with the catering staff for coffee, biscuits, and soft drinks to be available on each day of the examinations both for examiners and candidates. If possible, build into the time schedule a short break in mid-morning and mid-afternoon. Try to arrange a quiet, restful place in the hospital for lunch for the examiners and don't forget to buy some sherry. Finally, arrange for signposts to be put up around the hospital directing candidates to the appropriate ward, and alert porters and receptionists.

Examination day

Arrive at the hospital well before the examination starts. There will always be unexpected problems: the main road to the hospital may be blocked with snow; the coffee urn may have broken; the examination ward may have been taken over by decorators; your secretary may be off sick (the worst possible catastrophe); you may have forgotten to rearrange an outpatient clinic; or the key to the office containing the patients' scripts may be lost. There will be the inevitable last minute cancellations by patients and a few "disappearing physical sign syndromes." Always have a few spare patients in the wards (especially with cardiovascular and abdominal signs) who can be substituted. A round of the main wards the day before the examination can be rewarding and will put your mind at rest.

Try to start the examination on time as it is very difficult to pick up time if you begin late. When the examiners arrive, coffee and biscuits will promote a friendly start. Check the patients' physical signs yourself and then introduce them to the examiners; allow about half an hour for 12 short cases.

Have a plan showing when each candidate has to be with each set of examiners, and give the plan to all invigilators and to each examiner, so that there will be no confusion as to which examiners should be with which candidate and where. For example:

Examiners	1000–1100* Long cases	1120–1140 Short cases Candidate No	1140–1200 Oral
A and B	215	216	217
C and D	216	217	215
E and F	217	215	216

*Allow for 15–20 minutes' questioning on the long case.

Conduct of the examination

Ensure that the relevant instruments are available on a trolley in a central area and that the ophthalmoscopes are working. Candidates will also require paper and clipboards; have a few pencils available. Patients used as long cases should produce a urine sample but must never be forced to do so. Try to keep the long cases separate from the short cases. Patients who require fundoscopy examination should be put in a darker area if possible. I generally dilate the pupils; if this is done don't forget to constrict them at the end of the examination.

You will need one or more colleagues to help invigilate and to ensure accurate, synchronous timing and guiding of candidates and examiners. Registrars are a valuable asset for this and can help put candidates at their ease. They also find it a useful experience, especially if they can be paid a small honorarium. It is best to keep time from a wall clock in the ward that is clear for everyone to see. I usually give a half time warning and a warning two minutes from the end to examiners, as well as a final warning by bell or alarm—even if they say that they will time themselves—so that I feel completely in control. Sometimes a little gentle bullying is necessary to ensure that examiners keep to their schedules. (I have never heard of an examiner complaining that lunch came too early.)

It is important that all patients are seen during the examination. Keep a mental tally during the session, and if a patient is not being used inform the senior examiner and tactfully ask if the patient could be used when it is convenient.

When a candidate has finished never succumb to the temptation to discuss the correct diagnoses even if the day has ended. This is unfair to previous candidates and will often result in concern rather than succour.

End of the examination

Collect all relevant paperwork that has to be forwarded to the examination body, and thank all the patients and staff who have helped. If the examiners have left any sherry this may be a good time to offer some liquid resuscitation to the many staff who have helped in the invigilation.

Do not expect organisation of an examination to be a particularly gratifying experience, other than to give much personal satisfaction. You may be motivated by the proverb that "humility goes before honour" but you are more likely to feel, in Sir Walter Scott's words, "unwept, unhonoured and unsung."

Start in private practice

ANTHONY E YOUNG

I suspect that most senior registrars are appointed to consultant posts in the National Health Service with only the sketchiest of notions about private practice. This may be an encouraging reflection on their commitment to the principles of the NHS but it leaves them unprepared for private practice, and the best advice I can give for the newly appointed consultant wishing to enter this is that he should find an approachable senior colleague and unashamedly ask for advice about the practicalities and local arrangements. I was fortunate enough to have colleagues who gave me this advice unbidden, but for those of you too shy to make that approach the following broad observations are made. They are based on experiences in surgical practice in London and I accept that they may not be relevant to the practice of venereology in Wick or anaesthesia in Penzance.

Why private practice?

From the patient's point of view private practice entails the buying of a consultant's time. In addition the patient is expecting to buy comfort and convenience. Sadly, many patients believe that they can buy a "better" consultant opinion or a more effective operation privately and though I would like to believe that there is no difference in the opinions and skills available in the two different settings, I must ruefully admit that the current fraught and constricted practice in the NHS may mean that better medicine is indeed available in the private sector, even when the same doctor is concerned.

Overall the time factor is probably the most important, and after a few relaxed half to one hour new patient consultations you will quickly wonder how we do justice to patients and their diseases in the hectic NHS schedule. Adequate time is a pleasure as well as a necessity; it improves your clinical habits and sets standards that you should hope to be able to emulate in the NHS. Much has been written about the relationship between the NHS and private practice and it is not the purpose of this chapter to root around in the ideological detritus of the various arguments. For the moment the two exist in parallel, and consultants overlap between the two. The consultant's task is to make the system work to the benefit of all his patients and there is no reason why proper care of NHS patients and of private patients should be incompatible if the consultant uses his skills honestly and his time effectively.

It goes without saying that the private patient expects the consistent personal attention of one doctor, but it is a sad indication of people's perception of the uncertainties of the NHS that they will often ask at a private consultation, "And will *you* be doing the operation?"

Setting aside the time

Even a very busy consultant's NHS commitments will leave him some free time for private practice. If he is less than full time that extra time will be complete sessions; if he is truly full time he may need to find that time at the beginning or end of the working day or at weekends. Wherever that time is found it is best to structure it. Arrange a definite time of the week to see patients and if you are a surgeon arrange a regular operating time. Without that, not only is your orderly practice disrupted but life becomes difficult for your secretary and your family. Don't be coy about these sessions: they are a perfectly proper part of your professional life and should feature on your hospital timetable just as your hospital schedule appears on your private timetable. There is nothing more infuriating for NHS staff than a consultant who unpredictably dematerialises and cannot be contacted.

A particular problem for those who practice in London is grappling with the tight schedules required in the treatment of patients from overseas, who frequently come unannounced and want their definitive treatment today or tomorrow (or even yesterday). All you can do is fit things in as quickly as possible, at the same time exhorting them and their advisers to give some warning next time.

Private practice is, in essence, single handed practice: the patient is paying for you, not someone else. This potentially makes the taking of time for holidays and meetings difficult and shows how important it is to have an effective partnership or cross cover with your colleagues for those occasions. Partnerships also allow you to offer a comprehensive emergency service, something which is not widespread in the private sector.

Premises and secretaries

Private practice must be organised from some geographically fixed base. Traditionally this is the consultant's "rooms," the place where the secretary can be found and where patients are seen. Increasingly consultants see patients in several places, perhaps at home and also in private hospitals. That is all very well and it may increase the options for the patients, but for the colleagues who refer and for the patient on the telephone a central point of contact is vital. Even for those with a secretary, an answering machine is a great boon, preferably one that can be interrogated by you from elsewhere.

Few can now afford rooms and a secretary for their sole use. A joint practice—or sessional arrangements in a private clinic—is substantially cheaper and almost as satisfactory. Wherever you practise it is worth remembering that comfort and convenience are not just the private hospitals' concern. Your consulting room should be pleasant and tranquil to be in, for the benefit of both you and your patient. Choose your secretary carefully; she too should be pleasant and tranquil, sympathetic on the telephone, and endlessly patient with the disruptions that you will heap on her.

Full timers and those with small private practices may use their NHS secretaries but this is open to abuse, and the rules, remuneration, and hours need to be set very carefully at the outset and the agreement of the hospital administration obtained.

Many consultants employ their wives as their private secretaries and receptionists. A wife's salary is tax deductible under schedule D but to be so must actually be paid to her.

A fair amount of paper flutters around every consultation: notes have to be made up, addresses taken, tests and admissions arranged, bills sent. This inevitable mini bureaucracy works more smoothly if the secretary is in the same place as the consultation. If you are of the right bent a microcomputer might well ease these chores.

For London readers I should perhaps add a note here about Harley Street. Indeed not just for London readers. Otherwise sane men travel miles from hospitals in the outer suburbs to get to an address in Harley Street where they see patients who have made the same awful journey. I wonder for whose benefit this time honoured quirk persists. In fairness, however, I should admit that Harley Street and its environs contain a very talented and comprehensive set of medical facilities—though nobody should be under the illusion that the address guarantees quality, as any reader of the Sunday newspapers will know. The phenomenon of Harley Street persists out of conservatism and snobbery as much as for any other reason and I don't think that new consultants really ought to feel an obligation to take rooms or sessions there, certainly not at the outset of their careers, unless the romance of the Harley Street reputation really appeals to them.

Where to practise

Private patients still have the option of either a private bed in an NHS hospital or a bed in a private hospital. Hospitals in the NHS may lack the thick carpets and warm lighting of the private clinics, but make up with a wider range of medical services. Where you admit the patient depends on his wishes and his diseases. Not all private hospitals can cope with complex or severe illness and in dealing with these the full NHS team has advantages. Remember, however, that though such patients may be educational, junior NHS staff may resent time spent with them, and their efforts should be not taken for granted or abused. You should also consult the DHSS handbook, *Management of Private Practice in Health Service Hospitals in England and Wales.*

When a surgeon has another doctor to assist him at a private operation in a private hospital the assistant must be paid—and promptly. Some surgeons do not pay if the patient defaults; though this may serve as an object lesson in financial reality, it seems to me to be improper. When the assistant is the patient's general practitioner a fee is usually still expected though the amount may be difficult to judge.

Private hospitals are in general pleasant places in which to practise, and nurses are less stressed than they seem to be in the NHS. The quieter environment and the smaller scale of most such hospitals give them an atmosphere reminiscent of cottage hospitals of old.

Developing a practice

Britain's position near the bottom of the European "league table" of doctors per head of population guarantees that in the NHS none of us sits in the outpatient clinic twiddling his thumbs waiting for patients to be referred. One is led to believe that in certain well heeled southern county towns the same applies in private practice, but for most consultants there is the sobering realisation that in the private sector practice has to be earned not taken for granted. This is one of the virtues of the activity. Advertising for practice is not allowed beyond a restrained card to general practitioners and colleagues advising them that you are available and giving them your address and your consultation times; after that, like the man in the newly opened shop or gallery, you must just sit smiling confidently and wait to see what happens.

At the outset some patients will come, as doctors try you out; after that your practice can go either way—up or down. One would like to think that the progress of one's practice reflected the quality of service offered but it is of course more complicated than that. Social contacts probably count more than anything—a fact not wasted on those who, to the disgust of their colleagues, spend time and money developing social bonds with people with whom they might not otherwise bother to pass the time of day. Nevertheless, it is nice to think that patients come because they want to see you, and there is enormous satisfaction in seeing as new patients people who come on the specific recommendation of a patient previously treated. It is worth noting in passing at this point that though it is preferable for patients to be referred from their general practitioners or other doctors, as they are in the health service, there is no rule that says this must be done, and private practice continues to offer a convenient escape route for patients who feel dissatisfied with their general practitioner or local hospital. Most health insurance companies do, however, insist on referral being from a general practitioner.

There are two fallacies to beware of. First, do not expect to inherit the practice of your NHS predecessor. Very few give up their NHS and private practices simultaneously. Second, never believe what you are told about the size of other people's practices, particularly if they are vulgar enough to tell you themselves. Such claims are like fishing stories, and the magnification quotient ranges upwards from two times reality.

Money

We are all spoilt by being brought up in the NHS with a regular salary and hardly a care in the world about the money we spend on our patients. For this reason the financial side of private practice brings surprises for the newcomer.

The nice surprise is of course the extra income that it brings. The other surprise is the sudden awareness of how much everything costs. You see the bills for the bed and the blood tests, and if the patient is uninsured you must quickly develop a lean view of what is really essential for his care. Those few extra days in hospital can set him back £1000, the computed tomography done to document the lesion that you are not going to treat £300, the frozen section done so that the nature of the lump will be known tonight not tomorrow £250. Now try pricing unnecessary parenteral nutrition, fancy drugs, the endoscopies to watch an ulcer healing, and you quickly realise how prodigal the health service can be. The uninsured or underinsured patient brings with him a lot of anxieties about the cost of his care and it is important to spell out very carefully for such people the possible costs that they are or may be committing themselves to; indeed they may need to be persuaded back into the arms of the NHS. This is allowed. Patients may change horses in midstream, but only once in any particular episode of illness. Patients very rarely ask how much their treatment will cost, and the doctor is honour bound to have done those sums even if the patient doesn't ask. One colleague of mine produces written estimates like a builder. That is no bad thing, and incidentally one does not need to add VAT: doctors are exempt.

The financial side of private practice requires two things. The first is accurate and tidy book keeping; the second is an accountant. The new consultant who thinks he can manage his own accounts will, unless he takes an unhealthy pleasure in figures, find himself quickly out of his depth in the murkier corners of self employed income tax, schedule 4 National Insurance exemption, and rolled over capital gains tax. I doubt if many accountants inject their own haemorrhoids and likewise I would advise you not to attempt your own accounts. It is worth talking to your accountant well before the first tax demand appears as a certain amount of forward planning is needed. You may for instance need to set the end of your accounting year at the end of April, allowing an extra year's breathing space before the first tax is due. To someone brought up on PAYE the need to write cheques for the Inland Revenue on fees long since spent may come as an embarrassment. Thus from the start it is prudent to set aside, say, 25% of your private earnings in anticipation of a juicy tax demand. Although schedule D is more generous with allowances that the schedule E of PAYE, the costs of setting up in practice are by no means all tax deductable, so don't rush out and buy a new car.

New consultants may be anxious about what fees they should charge patients. This need not be a source of anxiety as in each geographical area there are fairly standard fees for new and for follow up consultations and the insurance companies issue lists categorising operations into minor, intermediate, major, and major plus types. In addition they settle the amount that they will reimburse for an operation in any category. There are ill concealed murmurs of dissatisfaction about the levels of these fees and their unbalanced nature favouring certain specialities. Nevertheless, insured patients reasonably expect to be charged what the insurance company specifies, and if you intend to charge more than that you ought to tell the patient in advance.

Conclusion

However small it might be, most people find private practice is instructive, stimulating, and rewarding—so much so that its enticements may be considerable—and it will thus do no harm to conclude with a warning about abuses of private practice that can too easily be slipped into. These include over treating, over charging, and over valuing your own skills so that you are tempted to treat in private practice those conditions that you would refer to your colleague in the context of the health service. Lastly, remember to be punctilious about your commitments in the NHS. Don't let an enthusiasm for private practice nibble into your NHS time. Your junior staff may not get any formal education in private practice but watching you will be their informal education and it should be correct.

Be an expedition doctor

JOHN DAWSON

There is no place for heroes in the conduct or medical support of an expedition. "Over-confidence is a factor that can lead to unexpected tragedy and failure."[1]

What is an expedition? Well, it could be a coach journey to Lourdes for a group of disabled people. It might be three days with a group of fit teenagers walking in the Cairngorm Mountains at Easter, or a new team taking over at a static observatory on the inland ice of the Antarctic. An expedition is a group of people, away from their normal surroundings, often without a fixed base. Being an expedition doctor requires you to foresee medical problems that may be caused either by the unusual environment in which the expedition will be travelling, or by pre-existing or predictable illness and injury among the expedition members.

There are four key points to consider when you start to lay your plans. These are: climate (heat, humidity, height); hazards (for example, isolation, decompression sickness, snake bites); help (local health care and casualty evacuation); legislation and regulations (mainly with respect to transborder transport of drugs).

Climate

Heat, humidity, and height are environmental factors that present known problems. Protection from their effects is fundamental to the survival of members of expeditions to areas with hostile climates. The *Textbook of Aviation Physiology*[2] contains an extensive discussion on factors affecting the survival of man in hostile environments. Although the book's purpose is to deal with the needs of air crew forced to abandon or land an aircraft, it presents arguments and figures that give a sound basis for the avoidance of hazard in planned expeditions.

Exploration Medicine[1] separates the medical problems caused by variations in climate into four groups. The groups can be described approximately as: hot-wet (tropical area with high humidity); hot-dry (desert); cold-wet (so called "temperate zone"); cold-dry (polar regions). Although the thermal stress of the desert is about two or three times greater than that of the tropics, both environments cause a heavy drain on body water, and the availability of drinking water ultimately decides whether or not a person will survive.[2] By contrast, the Antarctic ice shelf is a good example of a dry-cold environment while the Cairngorm Mountains in the north of Scotland should be classified as wet-cold. Over familiarity with the weather conditions of the "temperate zone" and specific factors such as inadequate clothing insulation can cause particular problems in wet-cold environments, and there are combinations of wind, rain, and low temperature that may make the Cairngorms considerably more dangerous than many parts of the Antarctic, which have lower temperatures but also a very low humidity.

Clothing acts as an insulator, preventing the loss of heat from the body by trapping tiny pockets of air. Creation of a layer of static air close to the body reduces heat loss by diminishing convection and conduction. If the humidity of the trapped air is raised, or if the integrity of the insulating layer is threatened by water, sweat, or precipitation, the insulation value is reduced. If, additionally, evaporative losses from the outside of the clothing are increased by wind, then a person may lose heat at a disastrous rate.

The problem of acclimatisation to high altitudes has been described in many books and reports. There is a good account of methods of avoiding and treating altitude sickness in the *Expedition Medicine Handbook*[3] which is published by the Expedition Advisory Centre (see below). The handbook covers topics such as expedition hazards, recommended immunisations and vaccinations, the problems of importing drugs into foreign countries, and clinical problems such as malaria prophylaxis and acute mountain sickness.

Hazards

The Expedition Advisory Centre, one of the founders of which was the Royal Geographical Society, is located at 1 Kensington Gore, London SW7 2AR, and the staff can advise you on many of the known local hazards that you may encounter in different areas of the world.

Once you have acquired information about the hazards that you may expect, you can plan a response to problems such as snake bites or fractures caused by a fall into a crevasse. Remember that the plans that you evolve should take into account the time for which you must cope before the casualty can be evacuated to hospital. Alternatively, you must reckon to manage from start to finish.

Machinery on ships and construction sites can be extremely dangerous. Even an experienced North Sea fisherman can slip on an icy deck and entangle an arm or leg in a wire rope as it runs through a block or on to a winch. The hazard is increased if machinery is operated by people with little training and a great deal of enthusiasm.

Injuries that are insignificant in themselves can be compounded by someone's desire to get on with the expedition without making a fuss. A swinging derrick may cause a minor problem if a crew member steps in the way and breaks two or three ribs. But if the casualty starts to take aspirin for the pain without telling anyone that he is also consuming a bottle of rum every day, the expedition is sitting on top of a burning fuse and a powder barrel.

Remember that a failure in the leadership of an expedition can put every member of the team at risk. On the other hand, poor selection procedures may subsequently present the leader with inadequate personalities or personality clashes that will make it almost impossible for the expedition to be led. Doctors are as likely to be affected by factors such as isolation, which can cause a great deal of stress, as any other member of an expedition.

Help

It is wise, before setting out, to establish the nature and degree of help that you may be able to summon once you have embarked on the expedition. Nobody but a fool will reckon to be entirely self sufficient when there may be the chance to discuss a case with a specialist in a relevant discipline, or the possibility of evacuating an injured or sick member of the expedition to an established hospital.

Time is an important factor which you must take into account when discussing casualty evacuation. If you know that evacuation can be arranged in 72 hours then your own plans for dealing with casualties should concentrate on stabilisation, the maintenance of homeostasis, and correction of those immediate problems that will not wait for three days.

Other questions that you must consider are: What communications will be available to you? (For example, where are the nearest telephones to the Lairig Ghru in the Cairngorms?) Will you have access to a secure satellite link? If you have to rely on high frequency (short wave) radio communications, will you be able to use radio telephony at all times or may you have to fall back on teleprinters or even Morse Code if ionospheric conditions deteriorate?

Once a communication path has been established, from whom will you be able to get advice? Many consultants rely on facilities that they take for granted and may be thrown off balance by a request for help in circumstances in which there are no radiographs, only the most elementary pathology, and a large, perforated baked bean tin filled with gauze into which to drip ether for an anaesthetic. Choose your experts for their common sense as well as their expertise, or get to know the specialists who have been approached by the expedition's organisers.

Doctors working in disciplines such as occupational health may be valuable sources of guidance because if, for instance, you are isolated at Halley Bay, on the east coast of the Weddell Sea, you may expect to have to cope with cases of carbon monoxide poisoning, as well as abdominal emergencies or insomnia.

Legislation and regulations

There are complex regulations controlling the exportation and importation of drugs in this and most other countries. Anyone wishing to take a controlled drug out of the United Kingdom must apply for a licence to do so. Licences and advice are available from the Drugs Branch of the Home Office, Queen Anne's Gate, London SW1H 9AT. Special arrangements apply for doctors who are accompanying groups of pilgrims to Lourdes.

Dentistry and other basic clinical skills

It is easy to forget that a dental abscess, or even an unfilled cavity, can become a medical emergency. Conservative dentistry may be beyond your capabilities, but you should learn how to extract teeth and recognise the common dental pathologies. Additionally, you should be able to give an effective local anaesthetic to allow you to remove or fill any tooth.

Analgesia and anaesthesia are important skills. If you can do nothing else for someone who is ill or injured, you can relieve their pain. If you have to carry out an operation under a general anaesthetic remember that you are not taking part in a crowded morning list at the local district general hospital. It does not matter if your patient has a heavy premedication and takes three or four hours to wake up after a general anaesthetic. He or she will be at less risk if changes in the level of consciousness occur gently.

Whether you are taking part in an expedition to the South Pole or working as part of a static geophysical survey team, stress is likely to create problems for you at some time. Work performance and interpersonal relationships may be seriously affected by a regular, excessive intake of alcohol. Members of static teams located in remote areas may use alcohol to reduce the stress of isolation and, paradoxically, the necessity to relate closely to only a few other people. Stress related failure in performance in one person is likely to throw an extra burden on other members of the team, in turn causing further stress. The *Expedition Medicine Handbook* contains a brief discussion of the psychology of small, isolated groups and the courses of action that may help to hold an expedition together.

Training other members of the expedition

Whenever possible, in a crisis you should follow routine procedures that have been established at leisure. Early in your preparation for the expedition examine the other members to see who might be able to hold a mask for a general anaesthetic while you operate, provide support at base if you are out in the field, or share the nursing of someone suffering an acute intestinal obstruction. Your training should aim not to produce a less skilled replica of yourself but to impart skills that will be complementary.

Sometimes the possession of such skills may be vital. In the case of the patient suffering from broken ribs, aspirin, and rum, the resulting haematemesis was handled with extraordinary ability by the ship's first mate, assisted only by a radio link to a doctor on another survey vessel. In the 24 hours before rendezvous was made with an Argentine ship carrying a medical team, the members of the crew caring for the patient had learnt how to take his blood pressure, had set up an intravenous line, taken and cross matched blood, and made an adapter to couple the ship's welding oxygen supply to the medical equipment. Although this case required procedures to be communicated by radio, it showed clearly the ability of people who are not trained health professionals to carry out complex tasks which can be literally life saving.

Conclusion

From a medical standpoint success on an expedition lies in minimising risk by scrupulous forward planning, and keeping a sense of proportion when times are difficult. People expect you to try hard, not necessarily to be successful. Despite everyone's best endeavours people do die on expeditions, and it is your efforts on their behalf that are important and that will be remembered. The care of people who are injured or ill should be shared with other members of the expedition. In your own personality a deep rooted common sense and quiet good humour cannot be overrated.

1   Edholm O G, Bacharach A L. *Exploration medicine*. Bristol: Wright, 1965:79.
2   Gillies J A (Ed). *A textbook of aviation physiology*. Oxford: Pergamon Press, 1965: 479–513.
3   Juel-Jensen B. *Expedition medicine handbook*. London: Expedition Advisory Centre of the Royal Geographical Society, 1987.

Broaden your mind about death and bereavement in certain ethnic groups in Britain

JOHN BLACK

Immigration from the Indian subcontinent into Britain occurred mainly between 1950 and 1970, but with a few exceptions the health services have not attempted to understand or provide for their Asian patients. It is possible, though undesirable, to manage an illness without regard to a patient's ethnic origin, but to be ignorant of the religious beliefs and needs of a dying patient and his relatives is unforgivable. Much distress and offence can be caused by lack of understanding.

Though acknowledging the importance of the religions of non-Asian minority groups in Britain, I think that difficulties and misunderstandings are more likely with Asian patients whose cultures and beliefs differ considerably from those of "Western" religions. This article considers only the three main religions of the Indian subcontinent—Hinduism, Sikhism, and Islam. It should be appreciated that within Hinduism and Islam, and to a lesser extent Sikhism, there are wide variations in attitudes depending upon the country of origin or adherence to a particular sect. A distinction should also be made between those who came from east Africa and those who have come to Britain direct. In general, Asian men from east Africa were businessmen, shopkeepers, or members of the professions and have a more sophisticated approach than their counterparts from the Indian subcontinent who have generally come from rural areas.

Hospitals, clinics, and practices in an area with a sizeable population of a particular ethnic group or groups should make adequate provision for them.[1-3] Lists of religious or community leaders should be available, and in areas where the numbers merit it, hospitals might consider the appointment of one or more of these leaders to a post equivalent to that of hospital chaplain. Ward staff should know that in some Asian cultures grief is shown more openly than is the custom in the West, and the provision of a side ward for the dying patient is a humane and sensible gesture.

The symbols of Christianity should be removed from chapels of rest and crematoria when these are being used by non-Christians; sheets used to wrap the body should be plain. Hindus and Muslims but not Sikhs believe that non-members of their faiths should not touch the dead body, and if it is necessary for them to do so they should wear gloves. Jewellery and other insignia of possible religious significance should not be removed from the body without permission of the relatives.

Hinduism

The majority of the Hindus in Britain come from Gujarat, in western India, or from east Africa. Hinduism is a polytheistic religion, embracing a way of life and a social system. Hindus believe in a supreme being residing in each individual, and the ultimate goal is the release of the individual's soul from the cycle of birth, death, and rebirth to join the supreme being. A person's deeds in his past lives determine his status and good or ill fortune in his present life, whose quality, in turn, governs his future.

Religious organisation

In Hinduism there is no supreme church authority and no hierarchy. Numerous gods are worshipped, each being the personification of a particular aspect of the supreme being. Most families worship at a shrine in their home, and attend the temple (mandir) for communal worship. The temple is in the care of a priest (pandit, a teacher) generally a Brahmin (a member of the highest caste), chosen and supported by the community. The priest has no parochial functions, but may come to the hospital to pray with the relatives of a dying person.

Imminent death

When death is thought to be near, the dying person is given water from the River Ganges (Ganga), and the family or priest read from one of the holy books of Hinduism. The priest may tie a thread round the neck or wrist; this should not be removed. Many Hindu patients prefer to die at home, and this should be respected whenever possible.

After death

As previously described, gloves should be worn by non-Hindus when touching or moving the body. The body is generally covered with a plain white sheet, though married Hindu women are often shrouded in red fabric. Normally the family wish to wash and lay out the body; this may be done at home, or at an undertaker's.

Funeral arrangements

The eldest son is generally responsible for making the funeral arrangements. All Hindus, except stillborn babies and young children (see below) are cremated. In India this is done on the day of death, but the formalities required in Britain make this impracticable; nevertheless death and cremation certificates should be provided with the least possible delay. Crematorium authorities should ensure the removal of Christian symbols for the service and their replacement by the symbol OM, signifying the supreme being. A well informed undertaker may be of assistance with the arrangements for the cremation. Ideally, the ashes should be scattered over the waters of the Ganges; but in Britain the ashes are scattered at sea, or over any large expanse of water; permission must be obtained for this.

Mourning

The family is in mourning until the thirteenth day after the cremation, when a special ceremony takes place.

Necropsies

Necropsies are not generally approved of, but if legally required by a coroner they are accepted, provided that the situation is fully explained.

Organ donation and transplant operations

There are no religious prohibitions against the giving or receiving of organs.

Termination of pregnancy

The only widely accepted reason for a termination is when an unmarried woman becomes pregnant, although there is considerable variation in attitudes.

Prenatal testing

Since the outcome of a prenatal test may be the advice to terminate the pregnancy, such investigations, whether invasive or not, should not be embarked on without a very full explanation to both parents. It should not, however, be assumed that termination will be refused. The concept of genetic counselling is not widely understood.

Stillbirths and the deaths of young children

A stillbirth is regarded, from the spiritual point of view, as no different from a child who has lived and then died. Stillborn babies and children under the age of 4 years (the actual age varies with local custom) are not cremated, as it is held that they cannot stand the heat of cremation, and have no awareness of their past actions. Burial can be arranged in a special area of a local cemetery. The formalities for the death of a child vary, but the mourning period and ceremony are usually observed, as for an adult.

Sikhism

The Sikhs in Britain have come from the state of Punjab in India, or from east Africa. The word Sikh means disciple or follower. The Sikh religion was founded by a Hindu, Guru Nanak, in the sixteenth century. Guru Nanak reacted against the excessive ritual, the priestly dominance, and the caste system of Hinduism.

Sikhs believe in one god, and Guru Nanak is revered as a man chosen by God to reveal his message. In Sikhism men and women are equal.

Religious organisation

There are no ordained priests in Sikhism; the Sikh temple (gurdwara) is in the care of a reader (granthi) who is appointed and supported by the community. The gurdwara may also be used as a social and advice centre, and for children's classes in religion and Punjabi.

Imminent death

When a person is close to death the family, sometimes accompanied by the granthi, pray at the bedside and read from the holy book, the *Guru Granth Sahib*.

After death

The Sikhs have no objection to the body being touched by non-Sikhs. The family usually lay out and wash the body themselves.

Funeral arrangements

The body is taken to the undertaker's by way of the family home, where the coffin is opened so that the dead person may be seen for the last time. All Sikh men and women, in life, and after death, must wear the five signs of Sikhism; these are: kesh, uncut hair (and beard); the kangha, a semicircular comb which fixes the uncut hair in a bun; the kara, a steel or occasionally gold bangle worn on the right wrist; the kirpan, a symbolic dagger worn under the clothes in a small cloth sheath or simply as a kirpan shaped brooch or pendant; the kaccha, long undershorts reaching to the knees, now often replaced by ordinary underpants which have the same significance. Sikh men wear their turban after death.

All Sikhs, apart from stillborn babies and infants dying within a few days of birth, are cremated. The ashes are scattered at sea or in a river, or they may be taken to a holy place, commonly the River Sutlej at Anandpur.

Mourning

The family is in mourning for about 10 days, though this varies. The end of mourning is marked by a ceremony (Bhaug) held at the family home. For children under the age of 8 or 9 years the arrangements tend to be less formal.

Necropsies

There is no religious objection to necropsies, but there may be some resistance to the idea from families originating in rural Punjab where these would not be usual.

Organ donation and transplant operations

These are accepted.

Termination of pregnancy

This is not generally approved except where an unmarried woman becomes pregnant.

Prenatal testing

Though there are no religious objections to this, the idea of amniocentesis or fetal blood sampling may be unfamiliar and require considerable explanation. In any case, invasive investigations on the fetus should not be done if there is no likelihood of a termination being accepted.

Stillbirths and the deaths of young children

The bodies of stillborn babies, or infants who have died within a few days of birth, are usually buried. The arrangements are similar to those for Hindu infants.

Islam

"Islam" means submission (to the will of God). A Muslim is a follower of Islam. Most Muslims in Britain have come from Pakistan, Bangladesh, or the Mirpur district of Kashmir (Azad

Kashmir); in some cities there are also quite large Turkish and Turkish Cypriot Muslim communities. The Islamic religion was founded by Mohammed who was born in AD 570 in Mecca (Makka), now in Saudi Arabia. Muslims believe in one god (Allah), and that Mohammed was his prophet or messenger. Mohammed is regarded as the last of a long line of prophets, including Abraham, Moses, David, Job, John the Baptist, and Jesus. The *Koran* (*Quran*) consists of the teaching of Mohammed, and this together with his recorded sayings and acts constitute the Islamic legal system (Sharia), there being no distinction between religious and secular law. However, some countries such as Turkey have a separate secular legal system. Muslims believe in life after death, and that a person will be judged by God according to his deeds, and may be sent to heaven or to hell.

Religious organisation

The mosque (masjid) is the centre for worship and religious instruction; it is in the charge of a prayer leader (imam) who is elected and supported by the congregation. The imam is not required to attend the death of a Muslim or to officiate at a burial, but is usually invited to do so.

Imminent death

The family pray at the bedside of the dying person, whose head must be turned towards Mecca; this may entail altering the position of the bed. The call to prayer is whispered into his ear.

After death

Non-Muslims touching the body must wear gloves. Normally the family wash and lay out the body, either in the mortuary or at the undertaker's.

Funeral arrangements

Muslims are buried, and never cremated. Burial should take place as soon after death as possible. The body is taken to the mosque or to the graveside, for prayers; women never go to the burial ceremony. Most local authorities provide special areas for

Muslim burials. As it is not always possible in Britain to comply strictly with all the Islamic rules for burial, some families take their dead back to their country of origin; this entails much bureaucratic delay which is very distressing to the relatives; but it is also the Islamic ideal to be buried in one's "homeland."

Mourning

The bereaved family are in mourning for three days after the funeral and visit the grave every Friday during the following 40 days.

Necropsies

As the body must not be cut or defaced routine necropsies are never accepted. Coroner's necropsies are reluctantly accepted if the circumstances are explained to the relatives, and safeguards are given that organs will not be removed.

Organ donation and transplant operations

These are rarely permitted, but there is much variation in practice. Refusal should not be assumed.

Termination of pregnancy

Termination is allowed only in order to save the life of the mother, but in practice it is increasingly used for social and medical reasons.

Prenatal testing

In exceptional circumstances, where prenatal testing (especially by non-invasive methods such as ultrasound) has clearly shown that the infant would be born severely handicapped, or suffering from a severe and untreatable disease, the parents may agree to a termination. Prenatal testing and genetic advice are particularly important in Muslim families because of the high proportion of first or second cousin marriages.

Stillbirths and the deaths of young children

There are no special formalities. In general, the body is given to the parents to make the necessary arrangements with the undertaker. It should be noted that for 40 days after delivery the mother is considered unclean, and may not touch a dead body.

Helping or counselling?

Nursing staff in particular can be of great help in advising bereaved and bewildered relatives on the procedures for registration of death, cremation certificates, and finding a suitable undertaker. The hospital chaplain may take on these duties and may be able to put relatives in touch with members of their own religion or community when no relatives are easily accessible. In discussions with some of the (male) leaders of the Hindu, Sikh, and Islamic communities I have not received the impression that there is a need for bereavement counsellors. It is difficult to obtain the women's viewpoint on this, as traditionally, and often for linguistic reasons, the man speaks for his wife. It is, however, often acceptable for another woman to talk to a bereaved mother. The Stillbirth and Neonatal Death Society* has often been of help to bereaved Asian families, in spite of the linguistic and cultural differences.

I am grateful to the following for their help and advice: Pandit Mathoor Krishnamurti, Bharatiya Vidya Bhavan, Institute of Indian Culture, London; Mr Jaspal Singh Bamra, Southall; and Hadji Haslim Ali, the Islamic Mosque, Whitechapel Road, London.

1   Black J A. NHS thik hai? *Br Med J* 1984; **289**: 1558–9.
2   Black J. *The new paediatrics*. London: British Medical Journal, 1985; 7–20.
3   Winkler F, Yung J. Advising Asian mothers. *Health and Social Services Journal* 1981; **91**; 1244–5.

Further reading

Henley A. *Asian patients in hospital and at home*. London: Pitman Medical, 1979.
Henley A. *Asians in Britain: caring for Muslims and their families; religious aspects of care*. National Extension College, 18 Brooklands Avenue, Cambridge CB2 2HN, 1982.
Henley, A. *Asians in Britain: caring for Hindus and their families; religious aspects of care*. National Extension College, 18 Brooklands Avenue, Cambridge CB2 2HN, 1983.
Henley, A. *Asians in Britain: caring for Sikhs and their families; religious aspects of care*. National Extension College, 18 Brooklands Avenue, Cambridge CB2 2HN, 1983.

*Stillbirth and Neonatal Death Society, Argyle House, 29–31 Euston Road, London NW1 2SD. Telephone: 01 833 2851/2.

Hospital Chaplaincy Council. *Our ministry and other faiths.* CIO Publishing, Church House, Dean's Yard, London SW1P 3NZ. 1983.

Islamic World League. *Funeral regulations in Islam.* Dar Al-Kitab Ali Masr, 33 Kasr El-Nil, Cairo, Egypt. (Obtainable from some mosques in Britain.)

Mares P, Henley A, Baxter C. *Health care in multiracial Britain.* Health Education Council and National Extension College, 18 Brooklands Avenue, Cambridge CB2 EHN, 1985.

Sampson C. *The neglected ethic; religious and cultural factors in the care of patients.* London: McGraw Hill, 1982.

Walker C. Attitudes to death and bereavement among cultural minority groups. *Nursing Times.* 1982 Dec 15: 2106–9.

Get a patient into a mental hospital

ANDREW SMITH

It depends on whether or not he is willing to go there. If he is, admission is as easy as getting a physically ill patient into a general hospital. Telephone the hospital, describe the patient's history and symptoms to the doctor on reception, and he will be admitted. This is informal admission and it is generally in the best interests of the patient and his relatives in that it avoids the stigma of having been certified insane.

Which section?

For the patient who refuses to go willingly, formal or compulsory admission is necessary—a much more complicated procedure because the Mental Health Act of 1983 has to be invoked. This lays down stringent admission procedures which depend on the patient's condition. If he is suffering from mental disorder of a nature or degree to warrant his detention in hospital for assessment (or for assessment followed by medical treatment), and he ought to be detained in hospital in the interests of his own health and the safety or protection of others for up to 28 days, he would be admitted under section 2. A patient suffering from one or more of the four forms of mental disorder specified in the Act—mental illness, mental impairment, severe mental impairment, and psychopathic disorder—would be admitted and detained under section 3, but only if, in the opinion of the two doctors recommending admission, he could not be treated at home or in the community. Furthermore, patients with psychopathic disorder or mental impairment can be detained only if treatment is likely to alleviate or prevent deterioration in their condition and help them to cope better with their symptoms. Such patients must be detained in hospital and cannot be treated as informal admissions.

Your first task as the patient's doctor must be to decide which section he should be admitted under, and having done so to contact an approved social worker or the patient's nearest relative, preferably the former. They are the only people who may apply for a bed in the hospital. Your next duty is to discuss the patient's case with the social worker, who will then interview him to satisfy himself that hospital treatment is the best way of providing the care and treatment needed.

Which form?

This is where the paperwork starts. There are no less than 15 pink forms, one for every contingency. Form 1 is headed, "Application by nearest relative for admission for assessment" and states that the relative hereby applies for the patient's admission, asks when the applicant last saw the patient, and states that this application is founded on two medical recommendations in the prescribed form. It then states, "If neither of the medical practitioners knew the patient before making their recommendations, please explain why you did not get a recommendation from a medical practitioner who *did* know the patient." Rather disconcerting for the nearest relative.

Form 2, which is the "Application by an approved social worker for admission for assessment," is more detailed, asks when the applicant last saw the patient, and says that the approved social worker has interviewed the patient and is satisfied that detention in hospital in all the circumstances of the case is the most appropriate way of providing care and medical treatment, of which the patient stands in need. It then poses the same question as on form 1, "If neither of the medical practitioners knew the patient before their recommendations, please explain why you could not get a recommendation from a medical practitioner who *did* know the patient." The applicant makes the appropriate reply and signs and dates the form. Form 3 is the "Joint medical recommendation for admission for assessment," on which you state that you had previous acquaintance with the patient before conducting the examination, and the second doctor—who is usually one of the medical staff of the hospital—states that he has been approved by the Secretary of State under section 12 of the Act as having special experience in diagnosis or treatment of mental disorder. You both sign this one and recommend that the patient be admitted to a hospital for assessment in accordance with part 2 of the Mental Health Act 1983. A similar set of pink forms refers to admission for treatment, rather than assessment.

There are three other forms for use for emergency admission, each headed in forbiddingly heavy black script, "This form is to be used only for emergency application." Form 5 is for when the nearest relative applies for admission for assessment, form 6 when the approved social worker is the applicant, and form 7 for the doctor's medical recommendation. Only one doctor need examine the patient in an emergency, instead of two, and he should know the patient, which means in fact that the patient's general practitioner should complete the form. The key sentence is that, "It is of urgent necessity for the patient to be admitted and detained under Part 2 of the Act. Compliance with Part 2 of the Act relating to applications under this section would involve undesirable delay." You must give the reasons for your opinion and sign and date the recommendation, which will ensure that the patient with this recommendation and the appropriate application form will be admitted to hospital. The applicant or anyone authorised by him, is responsible for getting the patient there—if necessary, forcibly in an ambulance.

Deal with a complaint by a patient

KATHLEEN M ALLSOPP

A complaint represents a perceived failure of a doctor to deliver the expected standard of care. This may be due to a failure of communication so that the patient's expectations are unrealistic, but a complaint may be indicative of a much more serious problem.

Complaint or claim?

A complaint is not a claim but may lead to a claim. A claim that a doctor has been negligent, if substantiated, may lead to the payment of damages. A complaint only leads to the provision of an explanation for the patient. Nevertheless, it is important that even a trivial complaint should be given proper consideration. Advice on the handling of a complaint is always available from a doctor's defence organisation.

When a mishap befalls a patient he or, if appropriate, his relatives should receive a prompt explanation of the incident. The information should be given sympathetically by someone of sufficient seniority to deal with a potentially difficult situation. There is no reason why an apology should not be made. Apologising should not be confused with the admission of legal liability.

Complaints about hospital doctors

A government circular, HC(81)5, gives guidance on which health authorities are advised to base their arrangements for dealing with complaints.

Minor matters

It is usually best for criticism of such matters as waiting time in outpatient departments or hospital meals to be dealt with immediately. Every effort should be made to allay a patient's concern. Conciliation not confrontation should be the aim, however trivial the criticism.

More serious complaints

When a serious complaint is received the consultant should be informed. All complaints should be investigated as promptly as possible. Most complaints concerning doctors relate to the exercise of clinical judgment.

A complaint may centre on a single consultation:

A child of 10 attends an accident and emergency department after a fall. He has cut his hand. On arrival the nurse cleans the wound. A brief history is taken and the senior house officer sutures the cuts. A week later the hand is suppurating and painful. Several large pieces of glass are removed. They came from the window through which the child fell. Subsequently the mother writes to ask why no one listened to the history and why no one took a radiograph.

On receipt of such a letter the consultant needs to ask the senior house officer for his comments. The senior house officer's notes are sketchy. He does not recall anything about a broken window. Now of course he wishes he had asked more. The child was nervous of needles so perhaps on reflection he had not examined the wound carefully enough. It had never occurred to him to have a radiograph taken. He writes down his recollection.

Having sought the senior house officer's comments the consultant needs to draft a response so that the administrator can reply to the complainant. The letter should contain an expression of regret that a complaint has been made. There should then be a factual resumé of what happened and why. In the case outlined above an apology that the glass was not found on the first occasion could be made. The consultant may consider that it would be wise to offer to see the complainant himself for discussion.

In many cases an explanation is all that is needed. If it is both informative and sympathetic the complainant may well be satisfied. The complainant may nevertheless persist with his complaint.

When a complaint becomes a claim

In the relatively simple sequence described above the family may believe that compensation should be payable for the unnecessary second procedure to remove the glass, and for the unsightly scar caused by infection. The doctors should consult their defence organisation if it is not already concerned. What was a complaint has become a potential claim.

Second and third stage of complaints procedure

Some complaints that do not become claims are less straightforward. The patient may have suffered a series of complications related to his condition. It may be difficult for the patient and his relatives to follow the sequence without believing that something must have gone wrong. On such an occasion an explanatory letter may need to be long, and may meet with further dissatisfaction however sympathetically and carefully it is worded. Such a complaint may be regarded as having reached the second stage in accordance with the provisions of the circular HC(81)5. The consultant should inform the regional medical officer so that discussion may take place. Sometimes it is still possible that further discussion between consultant and complainant may resolve the issue, but not always.

If the complainant persists, the regional medical officer may use the third stage of the complaints procedure whereby arrangements are made for two independent consultants to see the complainant and the consultant. This is intended for complaints which are said to be substantial but which are not at first sight likely to be the subject of formal legal action.

Complaints about general practitioners

Complaints about general practitioners are made to the family practitioner committee with whom the practitioner is in contract. The regulations for complaints are laid out in a statutory instrument, and strictly the complaint should be limited to allegations of a failure to comply with the terms of service, which are set out in another statutory instrument.

Informal complaints

These are complaints which are deemed not to show prima facie evidence of a breach of the terms of service. Many family practitioner committees use a conciliatory process, often in the form of a meeting between the parties with a lay person nominated by the family practitioner committee present. This system may work very well but it is not suitable for serious complaints.

Formal complaints

For a complaint to be deemed suitable for investigation under the formal regulations there must be allegation of a prima facie breach of the terms of service. Such a complaint must be made within eight weeks.

A patient's wife telephones the doctor at 1 oo am and demands an immediate visit: her husband is unwell. She claims he has pain in his side and his arms, and a cough. The doctor, after questioning the caller, decides that influenza is the likely diagnosis. In any case he knows of old that this particular woman is likely to panic. There is a further call at 6 oo am to say that the man is pale and sweating and losing consciousness. The doctor visits immediately but the patient has already gone to hospital by ambulance.

Some weeks later the administrator of the family practitioner committee sends the doctor a copy of the complaint from the widow. She tells the story of having impressed on the doctor the seriousness of the patient's chest pain increasing over the past six weeks and culminating in crushing chest pain radiating to the throat and down the left arm. The patient's widow is understandably bitter: when they got to hospital the nice young doctor there said that if only the patient had been admitted earlier of course he would have been alive now. Instead he died of a myocardial infarct within hours of admission.

On receipt of the administrator's letter the doctor should acknowledge it promptly promising a detailed reply within the 28 days allowed by the regulations. He may need to consult the patient's records, practice and personal diaries, telephone records, and visit books to check the facts. If a colleague or deputising doctor is involved in the complaint he should be informed. The respondent doctor may also be responsible for the comments from his deputies. The reply should pick out each comment in the complaint and answer it. It is acceptable to start with an expression of regret that a complaint has been made and to offer sympathy to the relatives if there has been a bereavement. It is appropriate to indicate how long the patient has been on the doctor's list and to give a brief outline of the relevant previous history including the rate of surgery attendance. Defamatory or critical remarks about the patient or his family must be avoided. It is important to try to achieve an air of calm authority and concern for the patient's well being.

In the case outlined above it would be important for the doctor to explain how he came to the decision not to visit and confirm that indeed he did put himself in a position to make a reasoned judgment, and that he had impressed upon the wife to call again immediately if there was any change or if she was anxious. However irritating it may be to hear that a junior doctor has been critical the reply to the complaint is not the place to criticise a hospital colleague. With a complaint to the family practitioner committee it is important to remember the question asked is not "Was the doctor negligent?" but "Was he in breach of his terms of service?"

The regulations provide for further exchange of correspondence and the complaint can be concluded after correspondence, but it may go on to an oral hearing at the direction of the chairman of the medical services committee. Doctors may obtain assistance from the defence organisations with both the written response and an oral hearing.

Complaints to the Health Service Commissioner

The function of the Health Service Commissioner is to investigate written complaints from members of the public about the provision of services or maladministration by a health authority.

The commission has powers to examine a health authority's internal papers and this includes the clinical records. A doctor faced with such an investigation would be prudent to take advice before giving a written report or oral evidence.

After investigation a report of the commissioner's findings goes to the complainant and to the health authority.

Complaints arising from private practice

A patient receiving private treatment will normally address his complaints to the practitioner himself. A patient who is declining to pay a bill because of alleged deficiencies in his care presents a difficult problem. To withdraw an account may be interpreted as an admission of fault, to persist after complaint as hardheadedly bluffing it out. Professional help may be advisable. Other complaints should always be answered. It may be appropriate to spend extra time—not necessarily at the patient's expense—to explain or inform.

Complaints to the General Medical Council

The idea of a letter from the General Medical Council strikes terror in most medical hearts. No letter from the GMC indicating that a complaint is being investigated should be regarded lightly. The temptation is to put the letter out of sight, but the proper course of action is to obtain the assistance of the defence organisation immediately; it is not wise to try and deal with such a communication without guidance.

Conclusion

However irritating it is to a doctor to be the subject of a complaint, a patient is entitled to a proper response. A lovable cartoon character is said to believe that a kiss on the nose turneth away much anger, but it would be prudent not to take the advice too literally for fear of complaints of another nature entirely.

Deal with problem colleagues

DAVID ROY

Relationships between medical practitioners, particularly in hospital practice, have always been complex, and attempts by colleagues or health districts to intervene when problems arise often lead to much bitterness and ill feeling. I do not intend to cover occasions when the law is concerned and the matter is dealt with directly by the disciplinary procedures of the General Medical Council, but rather to concentrate on the difficulties encountered by doctors who are mentally ill, including those suffering from alcoholism and drug dependence, and particularly when that illness directly affects the service that they are able to give to their patients. In addition, I shall discuss briefly clashes between colleagues, with particular emphasis on the blurring of issues between difficulties in professional relationships and questions of competence. These cases are much more complex than those concerning sick doctors.

Sick doctors

The medical practitioner's lot is traditionally perceived as a hard one, and few medical students enter their training without some idea, albeit minimal, of long hours on call, difficult life or death decision making, and, more recently, increasingly complex career choices with often dispiriting results. Many practitioners tend to be hard working, certainly ambitious, and to believe at the outset that they have resources to deal with an extraordinarily stressful way of life. Medical schools in the past, however, have tended to play down this aspect of medical practice and so have colluded with the doctors they are training and the profession as a whole in propagating the myth that a good doctor subsumes himself totally to the practice of medicine with disregard for personal health and wellbeing. The emotional needs of doctors have, for the most part, been ignored, and medical students appear to receive little training in these crucial matters. It is not surprising that doctors in general have not been quick to recognise the hazards of illness within the profession and the nature of these hazards, or that the methods of treatment and education deserve special consideration.

It is not easy to obtain data on the proportion of doctors who become mentally ill or develop alcoholism or drug dependence, and it seems that most surveys greatly underestimate the seriousness of the problem. Many doctors seek treatment outside the official information gathering services and it is possible that older doctors, who may be more liable to seek help for alcohol or drug dependence that has developed over some years, will be in a position to do so through the private sector. With the considerable increase in private health insurance this problem becomes more complicated, and the figures that are available from records of admission to NHS hospitals and referrals to confidential medical agencies must surely be the tip of the iceberg.

The commonest problem seems to be alcoholism and, to a lesser extent, drug addiction, with a variety of affective disorders also being diagnosed. Schizophrenia and organic brain syndromes seem to be infrequent. An explanation for this may be that schizophrenic illnesses tend to present at a younger age, and may account for some drop outs from medical school, while organic brain syndromes would tend to predominate towards retirement. Certainly all the evidence suggests that rates of alcoholism, drug dependence, and affective disorders are noticeably higher in the medical profession than in the general population, as is the death rate from suicide and cirrhosis of the liver. The presentation of these syndromes is no different from that in the general population; alcoholic doctors have the same general medical sequelae and psychological problems as anyone else. The only difference may be that, given the doctors' medical training, they are more adept at hiding the problem from their colleagues and possibly, because of their perceived stigma in receiving psychiatric treatment, denying it to themselves as well. Marital disharmony may be an important contributing factor in the onset of mental disorder, or indeed provoked by it, and medicine is not renowned as the profession designed to keep marriages harmonious.

Alcohol and drug dependence

The available surveys indicate quite clearly that alcohol dependence is the major hazard among doctors. This is hardly surprising considering the high status that alcohol achieves as a drug in medical schools and as a social stimulant in later life.

Quoted estimates in 1978 put the number of alcoholic doctors in the United Kingdom between 2000 and 3000. Given the increase in public awareness of problem drinking, the stringent campaign against drinking and driving, and the recent Royal College of Psychiatrists report on individual alcohol consumption which has resulted in a drastic lowering of the limit considered acceptable, there should be a reduction in these figures. Awareness of uninformed and uncontrolled alcohol consumption has, in the light of the alcohol policy recently formulated, resulted in the British Medical Association establishing a working party to investigate its own wine club.

Drug dependence in doctors is noticeably greater than in the general population and although some of the reasons given by dependent doctors are quoted as stress at work, overwork, and physical illness, detailed profiles of doctor addicts suggest that though they have fewer features of personality disorder than non-medical addicts, they have more disordered personality traits than the general population, and this seems particularly true for poly-addicts rather than monoaddicts.

In a 1967 sample the list of drugs abused was headed by amphetamines and barbiturates, with heroin and methadone trailing. The pattern of drug use has changed considerably since then and with the dramatic reduction in the prescription of short acting barbiturates and the greater control of prescriptions for amphetamines, that list must look quite different now, with the benzodiazepines and heminevrin possibly leading the field.

Depression

A recent study of 55 cases of suicide by doctors under 40 confirmed an excess mortality over that in the general population. There has, however, been a decline in the number of suicides by men, which is in line with national trends, but this was not evident in suicides by women and particularly so for young women doctors born overseas. They appear, on the evidence of this small but up to date study, to be at highest risk. A number of reported studies over the past 10 years have suggested increased vulnerability in individual specialities, with anaesthetists, psychiatrists, and pathologists being thought to be at greater risk.

The concept of "burn out" has gained currency in recent years. This syndrome can occur 10–15 years after practitioners are appointed to consultant posts and is often the result of waging the same battle over many years against a background of ever tightening resources within the NHS, complicated bureaucratic procedures, and an erosion of professional status. The rapid turnover of support staff with increasing difficulties of recruitment, a new management structure which many clinicians feel undermines their areas of influence, and the large patient load which is increasing in the face of diminishing resources, often lead to feelings of isolation, helplessness, pessimism, and inertia. Occurring at a time of great vulnerability, particularly for men doctors, this syndrome may explain the continuous, albeit reluctant, move of senior consultant staff from the NHS into private practice, and account for some of the increase in alcohol/drug dependence and depression.

Problems in treatment

Doctors make bad patients. They find particular difficulty in accepting the role of patient and there are certainly many professional tensions which arise between the doctor as patient and those who care for him, be they doctors, nurses, or others. The role of doctor as special patient further complicates an already difficult situation and may lead to early termination of psychiatric care on the part of the doctor. Although on one hand the therapist might be overindulgent or protective, the treatment given may also be cursory because of the reluctance of the physicians to pursue the therapeutic options as vigorously as they would with non-medical patients and this may result in poorer treatment and higher risk.

The National Counselling and Welfare Service for Sick Doctors

This service was set up as the result of an initiative by the president of the General Medical Council and the chairman of council of the British Medical Association in consultation with the royal colleges and their faculties. It is an autonomous organisation which is controlled by a national management committee and has appointed a number of national advisers who are senior doctors representing all disciplines. After an informal contact by the doctor in need, or a colleague, the national adviser, or a nominated specialist, may then contact the sick doctor making an informal offer appropriate to his or her needs and outside the district in which he works. No records are kept at any central point, and should the doctor need continuing treatment, records will be kept only as a part of routine hospital administration. This essential confidentiality will, it is hoped, enable doctors to take up various offers of help.

The Royal College of Psychiatrists has nominated 250 psychiatrists to act as counsellors in addition to 97 national advisers from various faculties.

The telephone number of the national contact point is 01 580 3160.

Sick doctors and the General Medical Council

Referrals through the national counselling service may fail or the situation may be too serious, and direct notification to the General Medical Council may be needed. For many years the only mechanism of notification was a formal one with a punitive referral to the council's disciplinary body, and health districts are instructed to have a procedure known as "three wise men" available whereby consultant colleagues, one usually being in the same discipline, are asked to make an assessment with particular emphasis on "illness." More recently an informal confidential procedure has been introduced whereby health authorities or professional colleagues (through the "three wise men") can initiate the screening of a potentially sick doctor by examiners appointed by the council. These medical examiners (two in each case) will report back to the preliminary screener on the doctor's fitness to practise and it may then be thought appropriate to impose certain conditions, such as the doctor accepting limitations on his practice while undergoing treatment. A medical supervisor, who may or may not be the doctor's treating physician, would keep the case under review reporting back to the preliminary screener and, should satisfactory progress be made, no further action will be taken. Should these informal and fairly benign procedures break down it would then be necessary for the case to be referred to the health committee, which may take statutory action by imposing conditions such as suspension. Only at this stage would notification of such a condition be passed to regional health authorities.

Health education and the medical profession

It is clear that doctors face considerable and particular health problems with attendant social and emotional consequences. Some medical schools have introduced counselling services for students, while others will only deal with the more serious problems when a student's performance is suffering. These necessary introductions are hardly innovative, and have lagged far behind the university campuses, polytechnics, and colleges, where such services are an integral part of student life. This may highlight a problem in attitude on the part of the medical schools towards the emotional needs of their students, who will be the doctors of the future facing the appreciable health problems outlined in this article. Medical students should be encouraged to take part in counselling courses, which will not only teach a technique basic to the practice of medicine, but enable students to engage in frank discussion of emotional issues. There is little discussion in schools of those aspects of medicine which do not appear in the textbooks, such as career choice and the increasing number of doctors failing to achieve their chosen discipline, management, relationships with colleagues and paramedical professions, being part of a team, and so on. Many of these issues will or should be part of specialist training in hospital, but the groundwork needs to be laid to avoid later problems. A straw poll among recent graduates from various medical schools indicates that they do not, on the whole, think that their medical schools deal with these issues satisfactorily, which is disappointing, particularly as pilot schemes have been introduced in some schools with success—although in others they have met with considerable resistance from the teaching staff and consultant body. The fact that most young graduates recognise the problem indicates that the schools are going some way towards facing it and they should be wholeheartedly supported in this.

Issues of competence and problems of professional relationships

In contrast to those cases concerning sick doctors, problems of competence have caused major difficulties in the NHS and there is considerable blurring of the issues in what can often become a cause célèbre, particularly where referral to the General Medical Council is not appropriate.

The source of this confusion is a document entitled *Disciplinary Proceedings in Cases Relating to Hospital Medical and Dental Staff* (HM (61) 112). Originally circulated to health authorities in 1961 by the Ministry of Health, this document remains unchanged since that time. The fact that the health service has moved apace, as has society, seems to have gone unnoticed. The document establishes, though by no means clearly, a series of steps starting from preliminary investigation for the establishment of a prima facie case and progressing through to a formal inquiry. These inquiries are formal and legalistic, requiring a high standard of proof, with many rights enshrined for the consultant under investigation, including the ability to comment on the proceedings, to make a plea of mitigation, and to appeal to the Secretary of State. In practice this results in years of delay and excessive cost to the various health authorities. There are currently approximately 40 NHS consultants suspended on full pay pending such inquiries, and this could add up to a cost of £4 000 000 to the health service. There is certainly a case to be made for reviewing this disciplinary procedure which benefits neither the doctor nor the service. Until we have a clearer system which has the support of consultants and health authorities, difficult and often painful cases will continue to arise in which problems of competence may be confused with difficult relationships and interpersonal problems.

Teaching districts and university based medical schools have different disciplinary procedures. The teaching districts' consultant contracts are district based and disciplinary procedures receive the attention of the district medical officer rather than being directed to the region, while teaching hospitals may direct problems through the university disciplinary procedure. Cases concerning professional conduct and competence in general practice will be directed to the family practitioner committee.

Conclusion

It seems that the procedure for dealing with a sick doctor has improved in recent years, although the reasons for doctors' greater vulnerability to particular health problems have received little attention, especially in medical schools. Where illness is not an issue, however, the position is clearly unsatisfactory and in need of change.

Admit that you are wrong

DAVID MORRIS

To err is human . . .

At one point in the preparation of this chapter I thought of writing to the editor, Dear Sir, I admit I was wrong in accepting your tempting invitation to write 2000 words on "How to admit you are wrong" because . . .

It sounded stimulating and challenging, but it did not prove as easy as I had thought. According to the *Oxford English Dictionary* wrong is "out of order, in bad condition, contrary to law or morality, wicked, other than the right or suitable or the more or most desirable, awkwardly placed, in a difficulty, at a disadvantage, *mistaken, in error (wrong opinion, guess, decision, hypothesis).*" These words in italics became my brief. I found it intriguing that 21 lines were devoted to "wrong" and 80 to "right." "To admit" is, by definition in the *Oxford English Dictionary*, "to accept as valued or true."

We have all at some time or another been wrong. The list that each of us could make would be interesting reading. The *Observer* recently republished part of an editorial, written 30 years ago over the Suez affair and condemning the government's action, which "incurred the fury of readers and advertisers." Some years later the late Iain Macleod commented, "You can be wrong by being right too soon"—illustrating the complexity of the topic.

Realising it

We each have our own set of ideas and values and we function according to them. We build up beliefs and convictions that direct our actions and practices. We all cherish our point of view, our allegiances, and the things we believe in. Our everyday life requires us to make choices and decisions, and though often easily and readily made, they can prove onerous. Choice entails deciding between different possibilities or preferences. Decision making entails making up your mind, arriving at a conclusion after formal judgment. There are those who find this so difficult that they drift into careers where they can easily pass the buck, thus avoiding both responsibility and authority.

When our concepts are challenged we instinctively try to defend them. When they are proved to be wrong the integrity of the system we have taken so much time and trouble to construct is threatened. How we cope with such a situation will depend on the circumstances and the implications of the mistake that we have made. There are circumstances when there is no room for doubt—a wrong dosage, an error of commission or omission. But it is not always precise and clear cut and without room for a different point of view. Extenuating circumstances can mitigate the wrong done. A house officer who has made a mistake may be pardoned if he had been up three nights running or had stayed on duty in spite of being unwell, not wanting to let his colleagues down.

What effect the realisation that we have made a mistake and are in the wrong has on us will be determined by what the error means to us and to those who may be concerned. Our reaction is part of our personality and character, our self esteem and confidence, but, above all, the degree of strength and tolerance that we have that enables us to be wrong and not be too seriously affected by it. How we feel in relation to others and what they think of us will colour the emotional effect of our error.

What kind of person are you?

The admission is another matter, but intimately connected with these subjective feelings. There are those who both realise that they have made a mistake and can admit it without undue difficulty. By contrast there are those who find it impossible to believe that they are wrong and cannot admit it. They will produce argument and counter argument and fight ruthlessly to win the day, revealing much of themselves and their emotional fabric. There are those who realise that they are wrong but share this realisation with no one. What an emotional burden of continuing guilt this must be. There are those who too readily and easily accept that they are wrong and almost proffer admission before it is due, which may indicate a form of masochism.

Reactions vary from immediate or delayed acceptance to denial, and there are varied accompanying emotions. For the experience is intimately part of our self esteem and our susceptibility to the opinions of others. This is an essential part of the process of reaction to approval and disapproval that starts at birth and never leaves us. Constantly and consistently we are influenced to learn about right and wrong, about truth and honesty, telling lies and cheating, and, above all, to cope with the mistakes that we make. These concepts are not easily acquired, for they are often accompanied by strong emotional overtones that confuse us and interfere with our ability to see the events in their right perspective. Why should disapproval and scorn, criticism and fault finding have so much greater effect on us than approval and praise, flattery and success? The pangs of loss, I contend, outstrip the joys of discovery.

In the practice of medicine, when errors are made we have to ascertain if the doctor took the necessary steps to acquaint himself with the patient's story and carried out the necessary examination. In the light of these, he arrives at an opinion which determines his action. No court would find fault with such a person simply for failing in the first two steps. What makes the mistake more serious and difficult to deal with is the risk to reputation and social and professional standing.

In recalling past incidents of being wrong, the one that comes immediately to my mind was to do with the first baby that I was asked to see on being appointed as a consultant. "A baby of 6 weeks old in extremis," said Mr Geoffrey Parker's registrar. I had never met Mr Parker nor had I been to the hospital before. As I examined the baby I could not for the life of me feel the tumour that I suspected of causing pyloric stenosis. I rang Mr Parker and told him what I thought and suggested that he operate on the baby. His reaction was explosive, which as I learnt later was typical of this extraordinary surgeon-parachutist to the Maquis.

"Right," he said. "But if you are wrong I shall never speak to you again, and if I am wrong I shall never speak to myself again." Strong words for a debutante to carry until the tumour was found. At the end of the operation he cut me down to size with, "Well, you can't always be wrong."

Experience the best teacher

It is said that a fool learns by his own mistakes and a wise man from the mistakes of others. How true is this aphorism? While there is an element of truth in it, our own personal experience teaches us more by direct involvement than wise counsels of perfection. There are instances when we may be wrong but are unaware of the error of our ways. It is only when it is brought to our notice that we are shocked to learn. A lot will depend on how we are told, who does the telling, and the importance of the error.

So where between the extremes of never being wrong and being too quick and ready to admit it does the well balanced healthy individual come, he who can see when he is wrong, accept it, and admit it without letting it take too much of a toll of him? The necessary elements are, I contend, a level of self esteem that can accept the human error to which we are all subject and the confidence in yourself to see the situation in perspective as being only part of the whole and not an entity on its own. Pride and vanity are always at play and vary according to the company we keep. It is a personal, very subjective, issue and has to do with how we feel about ourselves and how dependent we are on how others feel about us.

Practise audit

W VAN'T HOFF

Before dealing with the practice of audit I shall discuss the audit of practice and question the need for it. I believe that there is a need and I shall give my reasons for this. I shall deal mainly with medical audit as applied to hospital practice.

Auditing practice

Medical audit has acquired many synonyms and euphemisms, and one reason for the varied views on audit is the variety of interpretations of its meaning. It comprises not only the management and treatment of patients but many other things, including methods of and need for referral, the use and abuse of investigations or drugs, and matters such as talking to patients and their relatives. Some things can be quantified, such as bed occupancy, the time patients spend in hospital for various conditions, lengths of waiting lists, or waiting time in outpatients. A corollary of medical audit is that it should where necessary lead to improvement.

It is tempting for the purposes of audit to concentrate on problems for which numerical comparisons can be made between different departments or hospitals. It is often dangerous, however, to extrapolate from numerical information alone, because this leaves out what I consider to be one of the most important considerations, namely, quality of care. Quality is difficult to measure and therefore more difficult to assess. Often only the doctor and his patient may know the quality of care in a particular illness, and sometimes even they cannot truly make this assessment. If a patient has had treatment from a doctor who has been kind and caring, and he subsequently recovers, he will probably speak highly of the doctor and the standard of care. The treatment given may, however, have been unnecessary or inappropriate, and the improvement coincidental; yet both patient and doctor may be highly satisfied.

Although it is impossible to give a general definition, I myself regard good care and satisfactory management as the standard one expects a member of one's family to receive. Anything that falls short of this is unsatisfactory, and if there is anything that we can do to improve standards I believe we should make every effort to do it.

There is no general desire among members of the medical profession to adopt audit of their practice, and many conscientious and highly competent doctors do not see the need for it. Quite apart from the responsibility that we have as a profession to maintain and improve our own standards there is little doubt that the quality of care expected of a doctor has risen, particularly in the past 20 years or so. There are a number of reasons for this. The general public is on the whole better educated, and certainly more informed through newspapers, magazines, radio, and television. Much of this is good, but one disadvantage of the publicity given to medical matters is its concentration on high technology achievements. In an age where it is possible to acquire new kidneys, livers, hearts, and lungs expectations are often high and it is not always easy to explain that we cannot cure everything.

A question of numbers and education

Politicians responsible for the health service try to give the impression that all is well while at the same time making cuts that are affecting patient care. Their concern for efficiency sounds, and in many ways is, admirable. We should, however, remember that we are a service and not a supermarket. Efficiency is frequently equated with financial saving and, although elimination of waste is obviously desirable, we need to do everything possible to maintain the quality of our service. The doctor who requests fewer blood tests and radiographs than his colleague may well be financially more efficient but he may not be providing a satisfactory standard of service. On the other hand there is obviously no virtue in unnecessary investigation, nor is it desirable to have rules on how to investigate or treat various conditions. Nevertheless, education of students, junior staff, and colleagues by experts in a particular specialty can suggest guidelines for optimum management.

Education is an essential component of good practice, and improved training standards both in hospital and in general practice have contributed to better practice. Some doctors consider that staff rounds, clinicopathological conferences, seminars, and journal clubs constitute a form of medical audit. These activities probably do contribute to better practice but, although there is considerable overlap, they only form a part of medical audit. The rest is a conscious and deliberate exercise to assess the quality of patient care, to identify those parts of the service that need improving, and to take action to get that improvement.

Different attitudes

Not all doctors are happy about their management of a patient being openly discussed by colleagues. Some resent their work or methods of practice being considered, let alone criticised by colleagues. Sometimes this may be due to concern about confidentiality, but over and above this there is a tendency, sometimes based on professional insecurity, to avoid this type of discussion.

It is probable that in the clinical specialties in hospital more medical audit is performed in academic than in non-academic departments, both surgical and medical. This may in part be due to differences in work load and hence time available. But I suspect that there may also be a difference in attitude. Research is an integral part of an academic unit and, whether this be basic or clinical, the need to collect data, question results, and draw conclusions is common to both. The work entailed in preparing the results of a project either for publication or presentation at a scientific or clinical meeting is a further discipline. Inevitably conclusions and results may be questioned, and this leads to an acceptance that the work we do is open and not secret, and that we are prepared to stand by what we have done, or alternatively to accept suggestions or criticism where it is due.

Although it is impractical to subject all our routine clinical work to this sort of scrutiny, we should when necessary welcome opportunities to study aspects of the work we do in detail. It is common and very easy to be under a misapprehension about, for instance, your success rate for treatment of a certain condition. A proper assessment will not only give you this information, but it also enables you to compare this with those of your colleagues. There is always room for improvement and we should welcome opportunities for applying this to our work.

Practising audit

Until relatively recently medical audit has not been widely practised in this country. In the last century individuals such as James Paget and Florence Nightingale commented on the varying rates of postoperative sepsis and requested proper statistics to help detect and avoid these complications. In this century, however, progress was slow until 1952 when the Confidential Inquiry into Maternal Deaths was introduced. This has continued and has undoubtedly played an important role in improving maternity services. In 1969 the National Quality Control Scheme was started as a voluntary audit of chemical laboratories in hospitals. The scheme is now used by most laboratories and participation in it is required by the Royal College of Pathologists before it will accredit training posts. The scheme now also covers haematology and microbiology.

Numerous hospitals have cooperated in carrying out audit of radiology, looking at problems such as the value of routine preoperative chest radiographs and skull radiology after minor head injuries, while anaesthetists have studied postoperative deaths.

In surgery over the past 15 years a considerable number of studies both in England and Scotland have compared different criteria of surgical care, some within one hospital, others with many surgeons in several different hospitals participating.

In medicine the Royal College of Physicians gave a lead with its Medical Services Study Group (since renamed the Royal College of Physicians Research Unit) which was set up in 1977 by the college with the support of King Edward's Hospital Fund. This encouraged physicians to consider ways in which they could take part in medical audit. In most instances this has occurred within individual medical units, although in some instances physicians in groups of hospitals have cooperated. Medicine is more difficult to audit than surgery or obstetrics where progress or success rate can usually be measured after a specific event. Perhaps this, as well as the time, effort, and energy required has contributed to the rather disappointing acceptance of medical audit in medical specialties.

Clinical review

It may be helpful to describe the practice of audit in one district, the North Staffordshire Hospital Centre in Stoke on Trent. It comprises four hospitals, the North Staffordshire Royal Infirmary, the City General Hospital, the Maternity Hospital, and Orthopaedic Hospital, all roughly within a square mile, and with a total of 1340 beds. Most of the senior and many of the junior staff work at two or more hospitals. There are 32 physicians, and in 1979 they decided to start regular medical audit meetings. These are called "clinical review" and are held on the first Wednesday of each month at 5 pm, and last one hour. A complete print out listing all medical patients who have died is produced every month and this is sent to the chairman of the next meeting, who selects usually three cases for discussion. Each physician in turn acts as chairman. This spreads the load of collecting case notes and making a selection, involves all physicians, and helps to allay the resentment that could be induced if the same person always acted as chairman. It has also resulted in different types of cases being selected depending on individual interests.

The case notes selected are sent in advance to the consultant who had been in charge of the patient and either he or she, or one of the junior staff, presents them at the clinical review session. The chairman has usually chosen cases in order to bring out one or more points for discussion. These range widely, from delay over admission or transfer, indications and contraindications, for instance, for lumbar puncture in meningococcal septicaemia, need for emergency computed tomography, to appropriateness or cost of drugs used, care of dying patients, and so on. Radiologists, surgeons, and pathologists who have been concerned are asked to attend and the discussion is often wide, sometimes critical but I think always constructively so. The junior staff were hesitant at first, but now enjoy the meetings. They complement medical staff rounds which tend to be more formal.

To date the format of clinical review has not changed noticeably, although it was decided at the outset that it would be possible and probably desirable to do so. How much clinical review has altered our practice is difficult to say, but the participation of all the physicians and the agreement that cases for discussion are selected by someone other than oneself is a step in the right direction in the practice of audit.

Hospital practice review committee

Early in 1985 the medical advisory committee of the North Staffordshire Hospital Centre agreed to a suggestion that the whole hospital centre should take part in audit, and it was decided to form a hospital practice review committee. A chairman was appointed, and membership consisted of one person from each of the eight specialty subcommittees. Meetings are held monthly, and each specialty is asked to produce annually the report of a project concerning practice. These may be retrospective or, preferably, prospective. We have suggested that projects at first be relatively simple so as to show the practicality of the exercise. One such project investigated the wastage of blood ordered from the transfusion service for cholecystectomy. This has shown that some surgeons only requested crossmatching while others had blood grouped and saved. Only very few patients required transfusion and in many cases units of blood saved were wasted. It seemed likely that the second policy was probably handed down by consecutive junior staff rather than by design. A more uniform policy agreed to by all surgeons concerned could lead to a saving of about 1000 units of blood annually and around £18 000. An agreed policy may well spread to other types of operation. Other projects in hand concern infant mortality, and the results of barium enema radiology in outpatients referred for rectal bleeding.

The projects are not necessarily original but they are encouraging consultants to look critically at their own practice in comparison with that of their colleagues. At present these studies are being done by medical staff in their own time and it shows that a hospital centre with 125 consultants has accepted the principle of practice audit.

The future

I hope that the example that we and a number of other centres have set will encourage others to realise that it is possible to practise audit, and that it is constructive and indeed enjoyable. King Edward's Hospital Fund for London has recently formed a quality assurance committee to encourage this aspect of medical care, but for the practice of medical audit to become generally accepted it is essential that the DHSS as well as doctors accept the principle. Currently, so called performance indicators and implementation of the Körner report are concerned mainly with collecting information for management. It is essential that clinical details be made available at short notice, that computers be used for clinical as well as managerial purposes, and that administrative and secretarial staff help doctors obtain the information necessary for medical audit. Unless this is widely done I fear that practice audit will remain the province of enthusiasts rather than a widely accepted and routine feature of hospital work.

Standards are expected to be high in our profession. It is our responsibility not only to achieve and maintain high standards but also to be seen to be doing so, and by so doing, to improve the care of our patients. This is the reason for practice audit.

Run a clinical budget

K A M GRANT

One of the major changes that will take place over the next 10 years or so in the National Health Service concerns the ability to apportion costs directly to clinical work. At present the money available to district health authorities is split up into budgets which fund groups of staff such as doctors, nurses, or porters or which fund purchases of specific items such as medical and surgical supplies, drugs, or heating oil. These budgets are called functional budgets.

With the introduction of new computerised information systems it will soon be possible to relate the various items of patient care, such as laboratory tests and drugs, directly to a patient and also, albeit less accurately, to apportion what amount of time is spent by particular staff groups on the care of that patient. This will allow budgets to be apportioned to clinical activity. These budgets will be called clinical budgets.

What difference will it make?

The benefits of this are twofold. First, health authority members and staff will be able to see much more clearly how the resources of the health authority are being spent. With the present functional budgeting system it is possible to know what proportion of a hospital's budget goes on a specific purpose—such as providing nursing care, or buying drugs—and also to work out the average cost per hospital day and the average cost of treating a patient in that hospital.

Clinical budgets will show how much is spent on particular types of care, for instance, general surgery or psychiatry. The process will allow health authority members to see whether or not this matches their priorities. It will make the whole process of resource allocation much more open, and also enable financial information to be linked to the activity carried out by particular health care teams or indeed consultants. Health authority members will soon be able to see what returns they get for their money.

The second major benefit envisaged is that clinicians will be involved as the holders of the clinical budgets. The assumption is that as doctors are the major determinants of treatment, and thus the costs of care, if they are given more knowledge of, and responsibility for, these costs, then they will use the money more wisely, effectively, and efficiently.

Who sets the budget?

The budget will usually be set in January or February to enable all budgets to be approved by the health authority before the beginning of the financial year. The budgets are usually agreed at a meeting between members of the finance department, often in conjunction with either the district or unit general manager and the budget holder. During the meeting the previous year's budget will be reviewed and over or under spending discussed. Any changes in activity during the next year, including plans for development, are also discussed and then if possible built into the budgets. In most cases budget holders are asking for additional funds either to meet existing demands that appear to be under funded or to meet new projects that are considered essential or desirable. The meeting may very well end up as a negotiating or bargaining session. It is important at this stage to have your request for extra money properly worked up and costed. It is unlikely that any decision will be made at that particular meeting, as all the other budget holders will also have to be seen and their requests taken into account when the health authority finally decides what can be agreed to within the overall total budget available to it. The better you argue your case, the more likely you are to succeed.

It may also be that potential reductions in the budget will be discussed at this time, with proposals being put to you to reduce or change your budget. You should be prepared to discuss this. The budget meeting is, in effect, a review of the work being carried out by your department or clinical team and is the time in the year to discuss your work directly with management.

What does a clinical budget consist of?

This will depend very much on what local rules have been set out for the budgets and how far advanced the accounting systems are in building up clinical budgets. The developments will probably be incremental, and whereas initially you may have within your budget only a proportion of your activities this will gradually increase. There is likely to be a heading for the capital equipment and consumables that you will be using in the year and this will be one single entry in the budget. There will then be a heading for the staff employed in your department/service and then further headings for other items that you are required to "purchase" to carry out clinical care; these would include pathology, radiology, and possibly paramedical services. You will probably be allocated a notional part of certain facility costs, that is, the hotel services, patient services, and the nursing staff on the wards on which your patients are treated. It will depend very much on what local agreements have been set up as to whether or not they are allocated as a fixed cost or whether you have some control over whether or not you wish to purchase them.

What are the rules for running a budget?

These are contained in the standing financial instructions for the authority and will almost certainly be supplemented by a specific paper on the local procedures for running clinical budgets. This is very much a subject of debate at present with some clinicians suggesting that they should be able to determine both the quality and quantity of paramedical and nursing input; others suggest that this can be determined only by the relevant professions and that they should be merely apportioned to particular patients and to clinical budgets so that clinicians are aware of costs of particular treatment.

Who will help me?

The key person both in helping you prepare for your annual budget meeting and in running your budget over the year is the management accountant. He/she is an accountant working in either the district or the unit finance department who will be available either ad hoc or on a regular basis throughout the year, depending on how you are linked with the finance department. Make friends with him and use him. In particular, at an early stage use him to work with you in preparing next year's programme in advance of the meeting with the treasurer and general manager.

How can I monitor what is happening?

Each month you will have a budget statement which will show your progress. These are usually available three to four weeks after the end of the month to which they refer. They will show under each heading what proportion of your allocation you have actually spent. Under headings relating to staff they will show you how many staff your budget is programmed for and how many staff were actually in post the previous month.

Can I alter how I spend the money?

This is the main reason for having a clinical budget. Most districts have built in incentives whereby if you make savings under a particular budget heading you may keep them either in that year or in future years for alternative use in your department. An example might be the ability to keep and spend on alternative clinical care 100% of savings in one year and 50% for the next three years. You may save money by ordering fewer laboratory tests or altering your saving pattern and use the savings for the purchase of equipment or for going to a conference. This transfer from one budgetary heading to another is called virement. There are usually local rules as to how much virement can take place and to what purposes it can be put. In addition, most rules state that virement can apply only to planned savings. If, for example, your operating theatre was shut down because of legionnaires' disease you might not necessarily be allowed to use the savings to go to a conference in Honolulu. It all depends on local rules, and the main thing is to make yourself familiar with these rules.

What happens if I overspend?

In the end the only sanction can be to not let you hold a budget in the future. Obviously some over spending may very well be out of your control, and the important thing is to discuss the reasons for this, first with your management accountant and if necessary with the management in the unit.

Why should I do it?

The main reason for participating in this exercise is that you will have some control over your own destiny. You probably cannot alter the actual amount of money that you get to spend on your services but you can very much influence how that money is spent. If you do not then someone else will. There is in effect very little difference between running a clinical budget and running your own bank account—the only difference being that the sums are usually larger and it is someone else's money. It is ultimately good fun.

Keep up with the medical literature

DAVID P SELLU

Keeping up to date with the medical literature goes far beyond merely reading all relevant publications and attending meetings and symposia. It is equally important to be able to recall articles quickly when necessary, to cite references accurately, and to quote from them correctly. To make these tasks easier, you will need to do three things: (*a*) acquire and read the papers carefully; (*b*) make a note of the important information in them; and (*c*) store the references so that they can be retrieved easily.

Acquiring papers

Your choice of reading matter depends of course on your clinical, research, and general interests, and it will include journals, books, and conference and symposium reports. Good non-specialist journals such as the *British Medical Journal, Lancet,* and *New England Journal of Medicine* are excellent sources of general information, whether you are a clinician or a laboratory or research worker. Some readers find annual and biennial publications, which review and summarise recent progress, especially useful.

Many people read journals to gain general information, while some will be looking for material on a specific subject that interests them. You will have used *Index Medicus* at some stage for searching for references on a key word or topic, but it is well worth reading periodicals such as *Current Surgery* and *Cardiology (Rapid Literature Review)* which review many important papers published each month. *Current Contents*, a weekly publication, gives the previous weeks' contents pages of many of the popular specialist journals; scanning these pages will give you a good idea of the material published in the journals.

If you subscribe to a journal it will be in your personal collection; otherwise you have to read the library copy. There are several ways of acquiring papers that you do not possess: you can photocopy them from the library (you must observe copyright regulations); you can write to the authors for reprints; or you can simply borrow a work from the library. If you need to do a detailed study or review of a subject you should search computerised bibliographic databases such as MEDLINE or BLAISE but this service, about which your librarian will give you advice, is sometimes charged for and may be expensive (see also the chapter on how to do an on line search (p 83)). From such databases you will obtain citations of all your references, and, in many cases, abstracts.

How much time you spend reading new material each week depends on the time you have and the amount of reading you need to do. I devote about six hours, of which two are used for summarising the relevant papers and typing them into my computer.

Making a note of important information in a paper

It is useful to make a note of the following on a record card:

(1) The date on which the paper is read and the information from it recorded.

(2) The source from which the paper was obtained—whether a book, a thesis, a journal, or an unpublished manuscript.

(3) The location of the reference. The reference may be in your own or a colleague's collection, in your library, or in another library. If it is in a personal collection, it is a good idea to state exactly where it is so as to make it easy to locate.

(4) A description of the paper and of the work. This may be a case report or a general report, a leading article or editorial, a review paper, or a letter. It may describe or publish the results of a controlled trial, an original study, treatment, adverse effects of treatment, clinical pharmacology, animal experiment, or in vitro study, or combinations of these.

(5) The authors. The name of the author from whom reprints can be obtained is underlined (if a reprint is to be requested).

(6) The address of the institution where the work was carried out. It is always informative to know where an important piece of research was performed.

(7) Address for reprints if different from the address given above.

(8) The title of the journal or book in full.

(9) The volume number, pages, and year of publication.

(10) The title of the paper.

(11) The key words. The key words chosen will depend on your interpretation of the paper, but I choose as many key words as possible to ensure that the paper is not omitted when searched for even on minor key words. To maintain standardisation and ensure compatibility of my database with the general literature, I use only those key words which are listed in *Index Medicus*. Some users have developed a thesaurus consisting of key words from *Index Medicus* supplemented by their own key words on subjects that interest them.

(12) Abstract. This must be clear and concise and kept as short as possible. It must convey to another reader the main message of the paper and contain any other information that you believe to be relevant, for instance, whether it has useful references or is of historical interest.

Much of the information in (2), (3), and (4) above can be encoded to enable it to be written down quickly and to be stored economically. For instance, the source of the reference can be abbreviated to "B" for book, "J" for journal and "T" for thesis. The codes you use must be written on a master record card to which you can refer either when you are entering information or when you read the entry on a card, to see what the codes mean.

Storing the information obtained from the paper

This is the most difficult of the three tasks and it is also the most important. Your ability to recall the important message from the paper without necessarily reading it all over again will depend on how you file the information on the record cards.

If the total number of cards is less than 1000 you may well find it convenient to store them in a manual index system. If you enter three references a week you will exceed this total in just under one year, and by this time the number of references will begin to be too large for a manual filing system. You will have to consider a computerised system at this stage.

Manual filing system

How you file your references will depend on the way you wish to retrieve them. I recommend storing them under key words. You need a card box (or a separate partition in the card box) for each of the key words in your collection; the boxes are kept in alphabetical order. When you enter a new reference on a card you select the most important key word and file this master card under it. You should, however, be able to retrieve this card from the other key words and it is therefore best to create a duplicate card for each key word on the master card. You do not need to duplicate all the information on the card, but merely state where the master card is filed.

All the cards in each card box or in the same partition in a card box are filed in order, preferably in alphabetical order of the name of the journal in which the paper appears. Entries appearing in the same journal on the same subject are kept in order of the date of publication or alphabetical order of first author's name.

The advantages of a manual system such as this are the ease with which it can be created and the low cost. Retrieval is easy if the search is done on the variables on which the references were stored. There are serious drawbacks, however. If, for example, you want to look for all the references by a given author, irrespective of the subject on which he or she has written, you may have to go through all the references in each card box from beginning to end. Storage becomes a problem if the number of key words increases, and retrieval becomes equally more tedious. Some of those who have used manual systems believe that the system becomes unwieldy when the master entries exceed about 200. Errors in citing the references will always be a potential problem when the information is transferred manually from the card to another document.

Computerised systems

I do not recommend buying a microcomputer system solely for the purpose of storing bibliographic data. You should get a general system that can be easily adapted for other filing and for word processing. Considerations in choosing a microcomputer have been discussed in the first volume of *How To Do It*.[1] Apart from being able to store a considerably larger number of references in a computer, you can also retrieve them more conveniently than from a manual system. Thus, you can issue selection criteria instructing the computer to retrieve specific references—for instance, papers on a given subject written during a certain period and in a chosen journal.

If you do not yet own a microcomputer but are considering purchasing one, or if you have access to a microcomputer but do not have suitable programs, you may find it useful to consult the list I have given below of some inexpensive systems that have been used for bibliography. I have previously described how one of these programs has been adapted for storing and retrieving bibliographic data.[2]

(1) *Database management programs*

A "database" might best be understood in clerical terms by the words "filing cabinet." A database is an organised collection of data on a given subject or subjects such as, in this case, bibliography. The database will be composed of a single "data file" or several files. A file is a collection of records on a theme: the information on one of the cards described above constitutes a record, and all the records on a given subject such as "campylobacter" make up a file; and all the files together form the database. The record is divided into "data fields," each holding information on one aspect of the reference such as the names of the authors.

Some of the features that you must consider when choosing a general database management program that would be useful for filing bibliographic data are the following:

(a) the number of records that can be held in each file;
(b) the length of records;
(c) the number of fields per record;
(d) facility to write programs which create an easily used system, allow error checks, and enable one record to extend over many screens if necessary;
(e) password facilities to limit unauthorised access to data;
(f) ability to search for records on multiple variables, to create index files, and to use the system in conjunction with word processing programs;
(g) cost;
(h) ease of use and ability to run on a range of computers.

Database programs under £125

Cardbox (Caxton Software, £125)—Easy to use and suitable for bibliographic database management. Limited in its power to handle larger databases, but a more advanced form, *Cardbox plus*, is available.

dBase II (Ashton-Tate, £120 version for Amstrad computers)— Pioneering database management program, well tested and highly flexible. Good structural program incorporated to facilitate the creation of a "user friendly" system, but you will need help to learn to use it in this advanced form. Can be run on a variety of machines. There are also more advanced forms of this program, *dBase III* and *dBase III +*.

Reflex (Borland International, £99)—Good for the beginner; communicates well with other software.

(2) *Word processing programs*

One advantage of computerised bibliographic systems is their ability to move information from the data files into text files which can be incorporated into word processed text. This limits transcription errors, thereby increasing the accuracy of citations in your paper, book, or thesis. These programs can of course be used independently of your database program.

Word processing programs under £150

Bonnie Blue (Paper Logic, £99)—Low cost package with surprisingly useful features.

Easy (Micropro, £150)—Relatively simple and easy to use. Good features.

Perfect Writer II (Perfect Inc, £149)—Easy to use and menu driven. Good for the beginner.

Volkswriter De luxe (Lifetree Software, £99)—Excellent for beginners.

Wordstar (Micropro, £45 for Amstrad computers)—Leading word processing program; well established, but complicated for the beginner.

(3) *Computers*

The most important consideration in choosing a computer is

your program: get the computer that will run your programs economically. Fortunately, with increasing competition, the price of microcomputers is steadily falling. The new generation of Amstrad computers in my view offer the best value for money at the time of writing.

Amstrad PCW8256 (Amstrad computers, £425)—Price includes a printer and all cables and a special word processing program designed for this machine. The single external disk drive limits the user to some extent but the system can be easily upgraded.

Amstrad PCW8512 (£550)—As above but has two disk drives.

Amstrad PC range (Start at £500)—These machines will run many standard IBM programs.

(4) *Commercial bibliographic programs*

There are several programs specially written to handle bibliographic data. They are expensive and are intended for users in libraries, departments, and institutions who need to computerise vast numbers of references. One important advantage of these dedicated programs is that they can communicate with bibliographic databases such as MEDLINE and therefore provide means of obtaining a large number of references from the computer terminal installed in the department or even at home. My main message, however, is that there are many simple and relatively inexpensive facilities available to enable you to keep up with the ever expanding mass of publications.

1   Asbury J. Choose a microcomputer. In: *How to do it.* Vol 1. 2nd ed. London: British Medical Journal, 1987: 192–6.
2   Sellu DP. A comprehensive bibliography database using a microcomputer. *Br Med J* 1986; **292**: 1643–5.

Search the literature

JANE STEPHEN

When a doctor is faced with treating a patient for a condition that he or she knows little about—and certainly before he can write about it in a medical journal—he must first establish what if anything has already been published on the subject. In the jargon of the medical library world this procedure is invariably known as searching the literature.

It is in fact the essential first step for any new medical project, whether in the surgery or the medical library. Above all, the person carrying out the research—be it the doctor himself, an assistant, or the librarian—must feel confident that the search will be both comprehensive and thorough. So where does he start?

A good medical library, with a large stock of journals and indexes, is the first important requirement. The second is that it be staffed by a fully qualified librarian: he/she should at least be a member of either the Library Association or the Institute of Information Scientists. If the local hospital or medical library is unable to meet these conditions then without further ado the researcher should look for one that does.

Defining the topic and requirements

Once inside a good library staffed by a qualified librarian, the next step is to define precisely what the subject is. Are there, for example, any synonyms that cover the same topic? Any alternative spellings? Different transatlantic names? This process—which we will return to later—also often helps to clarify the subject in the researcher's mind, perhaps broadening or narrowing the scope of the study.

It may be necessary, for example, to put a time limit on the research—both as far as the time available for the research is concerned, and in terms of how far back in the search the researcher wants to go. If this is not decided beforehand the search could prove needlessly time consuming; it may be necessary to search the journals only for the past five years rather than the past 10 years.

And does the researcher want to read literally everything on the subject? It is often practical, for instance, to restrict the search to English language journals only. If a more thorough trawl is required, a decision must be taken beforehand to include everything written in foreign languages, and to pay translation fees where necessary.

It is during this stage that the librarian may prove helpful: he will probably immediately be able to suggest indexes or bibliographies in which the topic is particularly well covered. Or, to save the researcher time, he may be able to refer him to another library more appropriate for his specialised need.

Indispensable tool for researchers: *Index Medicus*

Any hospital or postgraduate medical centre library should have various indexing journals on its shelves, but all should have *Index Medicus*—going back, ideally, a minimum of five years. It is published by the National Library of Medicine in the United States, and is by far the most important primary index for any doctor carrying out initial research. It comes out every month, and at the end of each year a *Cumulative Index Medicus* is published bringing together the 12 previous monthly issues in sequence.

How should it be used? First the researcher needs to establish that it lists every medical journal that, in his opinion, is likely to cover the topic of his research. So he should start by looking at the annual list of journals perused by the *Index Medicus*: it is published every January and lists more than 2700 of the world's most important medical journals.

At this point a search can run into trouble. There are some odd omissions in the *Index Medicus* and for certain topics the list can be inadequate. A reasonably important and well known publication like the *British Journal of Family Planning*, for example, is not included, and for some studies that could prove a crucial omission.

The second stage is for the researcher to consult the thesaurus—known as MeSH (medical subject headings)—which is also published every January. This is the key to the whole *Index Medicus*, and in effect the index to the index. Thus MeSH lists all the possible words and groups of words that the researcher may decide to look up to cover his topic. He may refer to "old" or "geriatric," but the thesaurus will show him that the term consistently used by *Index Medicus* for the category is actually "aged" rather than any of these. The thesaurus is carefully controlled and revised each year, when new terms are listed and outdated ones deleted.

Because *Index Medicus* is an American publication the usage and the spelling differ from British style, as we have already discovered. So it is essential to check the British terms against the standard American medical dictionary. If the researcher needs to check on the meanings of any terms used in *Index Medicus*, he should consult *Dorland's Illustrated Medical Dictionary*. This is the standard work used in the preparation of *Index Medicus*, and once again no decent medical library can afford to be without it. It gives copious cross references—"See ..." "See under ..." "See related ..." and so forth—and by using these the researcher can easily avoid missing anything important.

How to use it: an example

Let us say that the researcher wants to find out everything published on sarcoidosis. From MeSH he will quickly find out that there are four "See ..." references:

Besnier-Boeck disease

Boeck's sarcoid

Pseudotuberculosis

Schaumann's disease

There is also one "See under ..." reference to:

Uveoparotid fever

He will also see that with the main heading of "Sarcoidosis" are other codes as well. He can then look these up in the second part of MeSH; here all the entries are conveniently grouped into family structures, hierarchical trees of related areas. So sarcoidosis is seen as being part of:

C15—Diseases, hemic and lymphatic

C23—Diseases, general pathology, signs and symptoms

By going through MeSH first the researcher covers all bases, and it is essential to do this and not to blunder straight into *Index Medicus*. A sensible way of proceeding at this stage is to make an alphabetical list of all the headings which it will be necessary to examine and to tick each one off when it has been seen. This also makes resuming after interruptions much easier. Then the researcher is ready to go to the main part of *Index Medicus*.

Limitations

If the thesaurus is used correctly with *Index Medicus* the use of Americanisms need not be a handicap for British users. Nevertheless, American titles take precedence in the listing and indexing; American journals appear first and others follow only later, so it is not always as up to date as might be desirable. Staying with sarcoidosis, the November 1986 issue, for example, includes American journals dated June and August 1986, British journals from April and June 1986, and Japanese journals from February and March 1986.

Alternative to *Index Medicus*: *Excerpta Medica*

Excerpta Medica is the next most widely used aid for searching the literature in medical libraries, but it is a second choice for most. It is published in Amsterdam, covers over 3000 journals—more than *Index Medicus*—and also includes abstracts, which many find particularly helpful. But, unlike *Index Medicus*, it divides its coverage into several subject sections; this can obviously make life more complicated but it can nevertheless be useful for a small specialised library, which can then subscribe only to sections of special interest like "Psychiatry" or "Cancer." Indeed, few libraries take all the sections.

Searching *Excerpta Medica* is very like searching *Index Medicus*; there is a thesaurus (*Malimet*) which you must first consult if you are to make a confident search. The time lag for inclusion of articles is longer than for *Index Medicus*, but the use of a printed abstract means that some researchers prefer it.

Other useful publications

There are other indexing and other abstracting journals, though many will not be kept in the average medical library. These include titles like *Biological Abstracts*, *Chemical Abstracts*, or *Science Citation Index*.

Another helpful publication is *Current Contents*, which is published in Philadelphia and consists of separate subject sections; the one most relevant to medicine is *Life Sciences*. It is weekly, and reproduces the contents pages of many other journals. Where this comes in extremely useful for the researcher is that it enables him to avoid the time lag of the indexes, and to be completely up to date about what is being published. It also enables him to see what he—or at least his medical library—is missing in the way of journals.

The search and after

Manually or by computer?

The use of computers for "on line searching" has meant that far more databases may be available to the researcher. Although manual searching can be slow and boring, however, it can open up new avenues of investigation that did not seem relevant when beginning. When only a few articles on a subject are required it normally proves the best, and it also has the advantage of being free to the searcher.

Keeping records

Anyone intending to publish their research will rue the day that they did not keep adequate records of their search. The method of recording the information is important and has to be correct down to the last full stop. Each journal has its own idiosyncratic method, the two most common being called the "Harvard" and "Vancouver" methods.

The most commonly accepted method of recording references is by using 5″ × 3″ cards, of the type that can be bought at any stationer's. The researcher should always take plenty of cards to a search with him, so that he can include even doubtful references which can be rejected later. Often it makes sense to separate each part of the reference, giving separate lines to the title, volume number, author's name, inclusive page numbers, and so on. (See the chapter on keeping up with the medical literature (p 70).)

Reading the references

When he begins his search it is sensible for the researcher to have in front of him a list of all journals taken by the library that he is using. Then he will know exactly what he needs to ask the librarian for; ideally he will complete his requests on forms supplied for that purpose by the library. Otherwise, as any librarian can testify, odd scraps of paper tend to get lost.

The librarian may be able to obtain photocopies of any required journal, and there are two main channels for this. The British Library Document Supply Centre operates one service, and there is also a network to which most local medical libraries belong. No librarian can produce miracles, and you should allow as much time as possible for the article to be obtained. No search can ever be rushed.

Useful addresses

There are some nationally important medical libraries which the researcher may be able to use:

British Medical Association
BMA House
Tavistock Square
London WC1H 9JP
Telephone: 01 387 4499

Royal Society of Medicine
1 Wimpole Street
London W1M 8AE
Telephone: 01 580 2070

Department of Health and Social Security
Alexander Fleming House
Elephant and Castle
London SE1 6BY
Telephone: 01 407 5522

Office of Population Censuses and Surveys
Saint Catherine's House
10 Kingsway
London WC2B 6JP
Telephone: 01 242 0267

Carry out an on line search

JANE STEPHEN

Put simply, this is searching the literature, but this time courtesy of a computer. The researcher selects his or her search terms—in effect key words—then asks the computer to match them with similar terms logged from indexed articles. If the researcher selects his terms carefully and knowledgeably the computer will then magically produce for him a bibliography of the desired reading material.

The procedures are basically similar to those of a manual search of the printed index, but where on line searching comes in particularly useful is when the subject is complex and difficult. It can also be much, much faster—taking sometimes a matter literally of seconds—and if carried out properly is exhaustive. Because the computer will neatly print the bibliography as well, it is usually more convenient and streamlined.

Not so long ago on line searching was invariably carried out in medical libraries with librarians acting as intermediaries. But now the development of microcomputers has meant that many "end users" can carry out their own searches from home, and so almost overnight what was a rare and exalted form of searching the literature is increasingly becoming commonplace.

Databases

Medical databases, in fact, were among the first to become available on line like this, and they developed from the printed versions of publications like *Index Medicus* and *Excerpta Medica*. But others such as *Psychological Abstracts* and *Chemical Abstracts* are also available on line. Indeed, some databases are only available on line, such as that of the Department of Health and Social Security. Databases are usually leased to host organisations that then make them commercially available. It can get complicated: different hosts may lease the same databases but each host may use different command languages—for example, either BLAISE-LINK or Data-Star—when searching Medline.

What is available in Britain

First, BLAISE-LINK. This group of databases is provided from the British Library Bibliographic Services Division, and all are medical or related topics; but the service actually operates from the computer at the National Library of Medicine in Bethesda, Maryland, in the United States. Some of the databases included in BLAISE-LINK are:
Bioethics
Cancerlit
Cancerproj
Health (planning and administration)
Medline
Rtecs
Toxline
Second, Data-Star. This system rivals BLAISE-LINK and is provided by Radio Suisse with Predicasts International Inc. There are differences from BLAISE-LINK. The files for Medline (*Index Medicus*), for example, are arranged in different combinations of years; as a result it is possible with the Data-Star host to make one search of the 20 years available on line, rather than the seven separate searches that would be necessary using the BLAISE-LINK host, as they do not offer that facility. Some of the databases available in Data-Star are:
Biosis Previews
BMA press cuttings
Chemical Abstracts
DHSS DATA
Excerpta Medica
Martindale
Medline

What you need

The researcher is linked to the computer by a telephone line. It is preferable to ask British Telecom for a specially selected line—a dedicated one, in the terminology—as an ordinary switchboard line may be disturbed by line clicks and noises and disconnections. But this is not absolutely necessary.

A special device to link the researcher's computer with the network computer—to enable them to speak to each other—is the second necessity. Such devices are called modems. Ideally they are integrated into the researcher's microcomputer, and a simple line and plug connects that to the British Telecom socket. An acoustic coupler, a device that fits around the earpiece of the researcher's phone and sends signals direct from it to the main computer, is an acceptable alternative if an integrated modem is not available or is too expensive.

Finally, to give the modem instructions it understands the researcher's computer must also have a package of software that enables it to exchange information with another computer, plus a working printer to receive and print out the information needed.

How to go about it

There are five separate steps in carrying out an on line search. First, the researcher needs to log on to the system. This is the step that establishes the link between the information and the researcher, and puts him in touch with the computer network—in this country the British Telecom Packet Switch Stream Service provides the link. Once the correct signal is heard the modem can be switched on or the telephone put into the acoustic coupler; then the researcher may be required to type in further identifiers and passwords.

The second stage is for the researcher to select the files on offer that he wants to search. Medical databases are usually divided into files which have to be searched separately, just as with the separate volumes of the printed index. In some cases, however, they can be searched in larger combinations. An example is that used earlier: the researcher may search 20 years of Medline in one go, or in seven separate stages, depending on which host is providing the service.

Third, the researcher should decide exactly what he wants to look for, and where. The terms used are usually to be found in the system's thesaurus, and although methods vary from host to host full instructions are normally to be found in a manual provided by the host organisation. Boolean logic is used by the on line systems;

this means, for example, that the application of "And," "Or," or "Not" quickly comes up with relevant references. Thus:

"Cats and Dogs" matches and links references to both cats and dogs.

"Cats or Dogs" matches references to either or both cats and dogs.

"Cats not Dogs" excludes references to dogs when only references to cats are needed.

Besides other facilities available, the use of subheadings as they appear in the printed *Index Medicus*—such as "Etiology" or "Occurrence"—can be applied to on line searching and this will pinpoint a specific reference and exclude unwanted ones.

Fourth, the researcher needs to print the results of his search. He can order his computer to print absolutely everything, with full and detailed biographical details; or he can request limited details, such as the title only or the title, author, and source. Once again, the commands used for printing differ from host to host. When no printer is available it is usually possible to have details of the search printed elsewhere, off line, and forwarded by mail.

And last but certainly not least, the researcher must not forget to log off. By switching back from the master computer to his own—and cutting off the running meter of expenses—he will see how much time was spent on line. This figure should be kept and checked against the bills that will arrive later.

Costs

There is of course the initial outlay for the equipment; then there are the running costs of carrying out each individual search. The cost of logging on to the main computer is the biggest expense, but the phone lines also have to be paid for in the normal way. In addition to both there may be database royalties and subscriptions to the host.

So an average search on Medline entails a local telephone call, and using about 10 minutes of computer time the search would probably cost under £6. The costs can be kept lower if you subscribe to only one host—either BLAISE-LINK or Data-Star. If the user develops expertise, and knows exactly what he wants and how to get it, he can cut down greatly on time.

Training for on line searching

Training is crucial in on line searching, because the better trained the user is the better the results will be and the lower the costs. Once trained, the user needs to keep in practice, too: some say that they need to do two searches a week in order to keep up their level of expertise.

The host companies usually organise short courses at which the system and command language will be explained. Then the learner will be given some "hands on" training, with an opportunity to become used to the equipment as well. Besides mastering the command language and thesaurus terms, it is important to understand the value of acquiring high quality bibliographical information from the master computer.

The host companies not only usually provide a manual describing the command language and giving details of files available, but also often issue newsletters and organise workshops; in this way the researcher can stay up to the minute with all the technology. There is another sometimes invaluable aid as well: most host companies provide "Help desks" which can be telephoned if the user needs assistance.

DIY or librarians?

It is only comparatively recently that anyone doing medical on line research has been able to do it for himself. But should he get librarians to do it for him?

It has to be said that if the researcher can do it for himself he is better off doing this. It frequently happens that when the task is left with a librarian, the doctor requiring the information is not present when the computer check is made and he is therefore unable to evaluate the information as it becomes available. Whether he is there or not, he must have full faith in the librarian's abilities, or go to another library.

Studies in the United States have shown that even when researchers use their own computer they still tend to turn to intermediaries for advice. They take longer, too, and are less able to modify the search requirements once they have started. Nevertheless the whole business of on line searching is expanding all the time and more and more new programs are being devised which should make it an increasingly simple task.

Useful addresses

Data-Star
D-S Marketing Ltd
Plaza Suite
114 Jermyn Street
London SW1Y 6HG
Telephone: 01 930 5503

BLAISE-LINK
The British Library
Bibliographic Services
2 Sheraton Street
London W1V 4BH
Telephone: 01 636 1544

British Telecom
Packet Switch Stream Customer Service Group
Third Floor
Tenter House
45 Moorfields
London EC27 9TH
Telephone: 01 250 8045

Use a word processor

LINDA JOHNS

The labour saving and efficient production of work has been the main reason for many people to give up their faithful old typewriter in favour of a trendy word processor. Now the latest technology sits before you, looking elegant and sophisticated: it's time to put finger to keyboard. But even the vaguest knowledge of conventional typing will soon show you that the keys on your new model extend far beyond the familiar QWERTY keyboard to left, right, and centre, many covered in abbreviated lettering or strange symbols. Pessimism about your ability to master word processing (almost universal at first) is strengthened by finding that even when the abbreviations have been deciphered the key may well not do what it says it should. This is because different systems use the same keys for different functions. So where do you start?

Getting to know it

Because of the many word processing packages available it is impossible to say, "Follow steps 1, 2, and 3 and everything will work." With each package using the same keys for different functions, templates (plastic covered cardboard, fitting over the keys to show what they do) should be provided and make life considerably easier. Look out as well for stickers that fulfil a similar purpose. These are normally found at the front of the manual along with diagrams and identification lists of the hardware—that is, the screen, monitor, keyboard, and printer. All word processors come with manuals. They vary enormously; some seem long and complicated, others compact and precise. Whatever standard the manual, it will look daunting—page upon page of instruction. It does, however, make life easier by listing the machine's functions and commands, explaining their meaning and the steps to follow.

Study the visual guide that lists functions in alphabetical order but also supplies a small picture or diagram to help understand the jargon. I have one piece of advice: try playing first with the obligatory "cat sat on the mat" or similar and, as with all typewriters, get the feel of the machine and its type.

The first command to master is printing. This is one of the easiest functions and also the best to start with because of the great sense of achievement which should spur you on to greater things. Anything more complicated, such as insertion, deletion, or the transposing of paragraphs—the one function that everyone knows or thinks a word processor should be able to perform—is definitely to be left until later.

One of the main obstacles to overcome in word processing is the jargon. Imagine how hard it is to learn a technique when the instructions themselves are incomprehensible. Some of the words will already be familiar to those who have encountered any form of typing before, such as pitch (the size of each individual character), header and footer (information typed into either the top or bottom margin), tabs, and proofing. Others will be new and will need to be learnt. These include:

Format line—The top line showing margins and tabulation points.

Cursor—The "blinking" dash pointing out your position on the screen.

Markers—Special instructions to the printer, for example, change of line spacing or insertion of headers or footers.

Back up—A second copy of the file on the same disk.

Defaults—The standard options the machine will provide such as margins, format lines and different keyboards.

The best way to learn not only the names but how they work is by practice: take each one individually and master the command as and when the need arises. Try to be systematic about learning. Too much too soon is guaranteed to end in frustration.

Getting to know all about it

Unfortunately, it is not possible to switch the machine on and have a screen ready for typing. "Booting up," as my machine calls it, has to be done first—a process of inserting different disks in order to get the machine ready for use. How this actually works will depend on whether you use a hard or floppy disk system, but the manual should give detailed instructions on what to do. It is important to remember that this is not a typewriter, and that immediate access to a blank page is not possible.

The next step is "formatting" the disks. This has to be carried out to enable the disk to store the information it is going to receive. It effectively divides the disk into sections in which the information is stored. Information can then be parked on the disk, and, because it isn't floating around, instant recall is possible. The information typed on to the screen, and then perhaps printed, must be filed away on to the floppy disk. Remember that, although the document has been typed on to the screen, the machine will not remember unless it is told to do so by a "save" command. Switch off the machine without having done this and the document is lost.

Now that the machine has booted up and the disk that is going to receive the information has been inserted, a "scratchpad" will appear on the screen (the blank page before it has been stored on to the disk) and, at last, you can type. Forward, backward, left, right, up, down—move the cursor around the screen with the greatest of ease. Make as many mistakes as you like; now it is possible to type over them, or simply wipe them out altogether. For all those who were typewriter bound with Tipp-Ex to hand, welcome to a whole new world.

Getting to like it

Now is the time to check your attitude before going any further. This is often the crucial factor that will determine success, failure, or plain confusion. The word processor is a machine, capable of seemingly endless tasks—still mainly to be learnt—that makes a plain typewriter look medieval. It does not think and it cannot read minds; it is important to remember these two points if you are to use the word processor to its best advantage. It will perform only as it has been programmed. Common sense, nuances of the English language, and poor grammar are things it cannot perceive. Work that looks badly set out on the screen will be printed just as badly, and spelling and grammatical errors will transfer likewise. Help is available for those with bad spelling. Dictionary disks can be used to check the document for errors; unknown or incorrect spelling is pointed out and the opportunity given to correct it. Beware, however, the American spelling disk; differences often make this exercise more trouble than it is worth.

Make sure that both you and the machine know who is master before you begin. Fear is often the main reason that many people shy away from word processing. With confidence and a more than average amount of patience most people can pick it up easily. I would recommend frequent breaks to begin with, especially when things are going wrong.

The manufacturers have included keys to aid your work, the greatest of which I found to be the HELP (sometimes labelled ESCAPE) key. Press this and the machine will show you what it is possible to do next as though you had an IQ of 10. A good key to find first. INSERT and DELETE keys, keys which produce capitals, bold type, centring, and justification are also on the keyboard. More complicated commands such as changing format lines, repaging, searches, and proofing (spelling check) are also there; locating them is advisable but avoid the temptation to do too much too fast.

Soon it will be possible to progress to these more complicated functions. But the word processor is not restricted to typing letters and articles. Many have a graphics monitor which provides the facility for simple art work, such as drawing lines and graphs. By changing the daisy wheel you can use different type styles and sizes for slides and overhead projector transparencies. Those machines with a graphics monitor will have a zoom facility too. The page and its contents can then be scaled down on the screen so that you can see how the type fits on the page, and can make corrections before printing. Baskets full of "previous attempts," not to mention time, are saved. Different colours for the screen background and type are also available and can be changed as frequently as you wish through the default mode.

Benefits of course

Courses are available to help you learn quickly, efficiently, and with the least amount of confusion and even though they can be expensive they can set the learner off on the correct footing. They teach the basic principles of word processing and even basic computing, enabling you to reach higher levels of efficiency much faster. Remember that such courses, lasting from half a day to perhaps four or five days, usually include any number of other learners, who will work and learn at different paces. It is possible to get left behind if you do not understand something properly: there is no time to waste when there is so much to be learnt. Nevertheless, having started my own experience with such a course, I would strongly recommend them. Prices vary according to the length of the course and the level of tuition given.

Some word processing packages offer training disks, possibly vital if you cannot attend a course. Insert them into the machine and they will take you through all the functions available, first demonstrating what to do and then giving the opportunity for practice, as many times as necessary until the user feels proficient and happy to continue to the next stage.

It is also comforting to remember the telephone help lines with experts to advise when a crisis inevitably comes. All that is necessary is to explain what is wrong; in most cases, through verbal instructions, the fault can be remedied there and then. In my experience all machines have fits now and again and it is reassuring to know that help is available from people who know what they are doing. One further note of encouragement: it is actually quite difficult to erase work unintentionally. I have to ask my machine to delete a document at least twice before anything happens.

No going back

The trouble with word processing is that the typewriter will never be good enough again. I say this from a user's point of view and not as someone giving work and being presented with the finished article. The electronic typewriter may produce as good a finished article, but I would never choose to go back to the typewriter because the word processor saves so much retyping of documents, especially when a perfect copy is needed.

Patience, practice, and perseverance are necessary at the start, but the rewards of the word processor far outweigh the time and effort spent in learning how to use it. And in the final analysis there is not only the satisfaction of seeing the words written on the paper but the actual enjoyment in getting them there.

Use electronic mail

MICHAEL S BUCKINGHAM

The National Health Service is a large user of the Post Office. New technology in the form of word processors linked by the telephone system may result in letters being replaced by electronic mail. What follows is based on my own experience of the introduction of such a system into a district general hospital.

Introduction

Information may be transmitted from one person to another in a number of ways. Talking face to face is informative, direct, and immediate but may not be convenient. Talking by telephone is also immediate but is slightly less informative and may entail delay while the second party is located. Letter writing is much slower but has the advantage of providing "hard copy" which may be filed and used for future reference. This is important for continuing patient management and for legal purposes. Good overall communication between hospital and community depends on a combination of these three systems of exchanging information.

Changes in the office

In the past, many referrals of patients were made by handwritten letter. Unfortunately the legibility of handwriting is variable, and so most letters are now typewritten, which is also faster. Typewriters have improved over the years from the heavy manual machines to electric typewriters and electronic typewriters with limited text editing facilities. The most important recent development has been the word processor, consisting of a visual display unit, a typewriter type keyboard with integral computer facility, and a printer. The word processor may be used as a conventional typewriter but, depending on the capacity of the computer, a large number of additional facilities are available such as text editing, data storage and retrieval, formation of letters, spelling checks, list processing, and text duplication. In many offices the major advantages of a word processor over a typewriter are that documents may be typed and subsequently edited without having to be retyped and that many identical "top copies" of a document may be produced from only one typing.

The word processor is therefore a desk top computer designed for office use. It does not, however, have to be an isolated unit. Because the machine can retain the information typed into it this information can be transmitted to a second word processor. A suitable communication network is the British Telecom telephone system, and as long as a suitable connection can be made word processors can be made to communicate by telephone. Documents may thus be prepared in one office and transmitted by telephone to another office, the document being reproduced on the recipient word processor's screen or printer. The transmission of information in this way, without paper being physically moved from place to place, is known as electronic mail. The principal advantage of electronic mail is that information is transmitted instantly and directly from the point of origin to the recipient. As far as hospitals are concerned this avoids the inevitable delay incurred in sending letters through the internal mail system and subsequently through the Post Office. (This may take up to a week or so while the electronic mail is received almost immediately after dispatch.)

A number of electronic mail systems are already in widespread use. The telex system (short for *tele*printer *ex*change) has been used for many years. This is a text orientated system and is similar to the telephone system but with teleprinter rather than audible signals. It transmits signals at the rate of 50 bits/second or approximately 6.6 characters a second, and, with teleprinters that are a combination of a keyboard and printer, provides a paper record for both sender and recipient. Nevertheless, useful though it is, telex is relatively slow and not very versatile. A development of telex called teletex—as distinct from teletext, which is a system for receiving broadcast information on specifically modified television receivers—has recently been established. This new system transmits at 2400 bits/second and so is considerably faster than telex. Because information is transmitted from one computer memory to another, using a word processor rather than a teleprinter, messages may be received without interrupting other work already being performed on the equipment. Teletex can also tie up with other word processor functions so that a highly flexible international telecommunication system will ultimately become available. This system is, however, very elaborate and expensive and best suited for large international corporations.

For the purposes of electronic mail within a health district a similar though less elaborate electronic system may be established. If such a system is to be comprehensive, terminals need to be sited throughout the district general hospital, in any outlying hospitals, and in the general practitioners' surgeries and health centres in the district. Any terminal will then be able to communicate with any other at any time. As well as being used as an electronic mailing system between the hospital and community, there may of course be communication between terminals within the hospital. This may be particularly helpful if it provides access to the pathology department's computerised records. Results of investigations will then be readily available, night or day, without any need to interrupt the laboratory's work or wait for the result to be found.

Using the system

The Winchester Health District is in the process of introducing the British Telecom Merlin business system. Each terminal consists of a simple microcomputer with a printer but no disk store. The computer terminal has a built in coupler that connects it to the telephone system. The computer may be programmed to store up to 10 master copies of forms which may be used, for example, for hospital discharge summaries. When completed such a form may be sent to as many destinations as wanted.

The visual display unit (VDU) consists of a small monitor screen divided into two parts. The upper part displays the document to be prepared, either a letter or memo, or in a programmed form that may be selected and completed. Twenty five lines of typing space are available on screen with a screen width of 80 characters. The prepared document is typed on to paper with 52 lines per page. The text may be moved line by line, in 20 line blocks, or in a complete 52 line page, so that documents may be reviewed and edited.

The lower screen consists of 5 lines displaying the various commands available to the operator (the "menu") which allow such operations as copying, editing, printing, or dispatching.

If a document is to be dispatched the telephone number of the recipient is typed on the monitor, and the computer then stores the document for automatic sending. A limited number of messages may be stored at any one time and there may be some delay if the recipient's number is engaged. The terminal will attempt to transmit the message five times within an hour. If it fails it prints out the entire message on the sender's printer to draw attention to the failure. The sender may then make further attempts to transmit the message at a more suitable time or, as a last resort, may send the printed message by post.

The hospital terminals may also be used to receive communications from general practitioners either items of information or formal referral letters. Letters may be personalised by being directed to an individual, and an electronic "signature" may be applied. This takes the form of a personal identity number which is known only to the person concerned and which does not appear on the VDU screen. Once entered from the keyboard the document is secured and no further editing is possible.

Privacy of information transmitted by electronic mail should not be a problem in a system of limited size such as that used by a district health authority although care must be taken to ensure that the information is directed accurately. Interception seems unlikely but if information is particularly sensitive then it may be sent by post, appropriately marked in the traditional way, or delivered personally.

Word processors such as the Merlin system can also be used for collecting hospital statistics. This must be reported to regional health authorities and the DHSS according to the recommendations of the Steering Committee of the Health Services Information (Korner information). Information dispatched from the hospital on prepared forms may also be directed to the hospital computer for storage and analysis.

Conclusion

When new technology is introduced there is always some degree of resistance from those who have to use it. In addition the operator will attempt to use the new equipment in the same way as the old. A change such as that from typewriter to word processor will result in the new equipment being substantially underused, so wasting many useful features. Staff must be adequately trained before such technology is installed or used. This is essential both for getting the best use out of the equipment and for maintaining good staff morale.

I thank the library staff at the Royal Hampshire County Hospital for their help in providing the background for this article, and my wife Hazel who typed the article on her word processor. It was delivered to the *BMJ* by post.

Make a video tape

PETER CULL

Video recordings have become a popular and accepted tool of record, analysis, and communication in medicine and they vary from the relatively simple, unedited demonstration of the clinical examination of a patient—which to make may need just one camera and a single operator—to a full scale teaching production involving many staff, studio and location work, multiple cameras, complex editing with insertion of graphics, film and animation sequences, over dubbed narration, and music. At each point in this spectrum, the technical and creative requirements are very different and so in this short article it is possible only to consider some general points. For those who, having read it and pondered the implications, wish to proceed further there are some excellent reference works available and these are listed below.

Improvements in video technology have taken place at a remarkable pace in recent years, and while quality and versatility have risen costs have come down. Furthermore, cameras and recorders are now so simple to operate that no amateurs need be deterred from using this excellent medium, providing, that is, that they recognise their own creative limitations and that of their equipment, and are prepared to invest the necessary time and effort.

The technical, production, and creative elments of video production are inseparable so I shall discuss them together.

Video formats

There are several video recording formats currently in use; the two most popular in the amateur/professional range are VHS and U-Matic, though others are fast developing. Both of these are cassette tape systems; VHS, using $\frac{1}{2}''$ recording tape, is the cheaper whereas U-Matic, which uses $\frac{3}{4}''$ tape, is mainly used by professionals. Generally speaking the wider the tape the higher the quality of recording and this is particularly important when tapes need to be edited or copied as each rerecording results in a loss of quality.

It is perhaps worth mentioning here that in addition to various formats there are also three different television broadcast standards in the world. In Britain and most European countries the PAL standard is used but both France and the USA among others use different standards. As a result a video tape made in Britain cannot be replayed in a country operating on a different standard unless the relevant equipment is available or the tape is copied in the appropriate standard.

Recorders

Irrespective of the format employed, the video recorder is the key element in the equipment, and it is worth spending a bit more to gain reliability and obtain the best results. It is advisable to choose a professional or industrial recorder with an "Edit" facility which ensures that recordings begin with a clean cut picture rather than a broken image that takes time to settle down (the use of editing in compiling a programme will be discussed later). Battery driven portable recorders with built in playback facilities are available in both formats and some recorders are now actually incorporated in the camera body itself—the so called Cam-corders. Portable equipment is particularly useful for a one man operation and in locations remote from a power source, or where trailing power, camera, and sound cables are a nuisance or dangerous. It is worth bearing in mind that when making recordings in sensitive situations—for example, clinical interviews and examinations, performance evaluation, role play etc—the less obtrusive the equipment the less alarming or distracting it is for the participant, and a better, less selfconscious performance will be obtained.

Cameras

Any video camera will work with any recording format and your choice will depend largely on the available finance which in turn dictates quality and the degree of versatility. Colour cameras based on cathode ray tubes can be divided into two basic types: single tube, where the colour information in the three primary colours is separated by means of filters on a single cathode ray tube; and three tube cameras in which a separate tube is devoted to each of the primary colours. A three tube camera is usually larger, heavier, and more expensive, but produces pictures of a much higher quality. Another type of microchip camera now in process of evolution operates without tubes—the CCD camera. This has many potential advantages and is a development worth following for semiprofessional users.

There are other factors to consider when choosing a camera: an automatic focusing facility can be useful for the one man operation, but there are disadvantages such as the fact that the point of focus must always remain in the centre of the frame, thus severely restricting picture composition; the zoom facility allowing a smooth transition from wide angle to close up view is an essential, and an automatic aperture control which adjusts the quantity of light entering the lens is extremely useful; high sensitivity will permit the camera to be used with the minimum of additional lighting and the so called low light cameras will operate with reasonable efficiency in a well lit room. This is particularly valuable in a medical environment, where banks of television lights can be both distracting and uncomfortable for patients and inconvenient for the operator to install on location in wards etc. The facility for synchronisation with other cameras may be useful and this is considered in the subsequent section.

Small, lightweight cameras can be hand held which is sometimes an advantage, but every vibration is magnified in the picture and this can be a severe distraction. Whenever possible, therefore, the camera should be mounted on a firm tripod.

One or more cameras?

Pictures captured from a single, unchanging camera viewpoint usually lack interest. The judicious use of the zoom facility and panning between two participants, for example, can improve the presentation; even so, too many repetitive movements of this kind can be disturbing and it is often impossible to establish a viewpoint from which every action and detail can be adequately observed. In such circumstances you need to consider the use of additional cameras covering the scene from different viewpoints and cutting between them.

This not only raises the financial considerations of additional equipment but also the implications of additional personnel needed to operate it—the minimum number of operators required in a two camera production is three. All the cameras used must be capable of being electronically synchronised with each other and the images from each fed to individual monitors for the purposes of selection by the producer/recordist. The images from the monitors are fed into a mixing unit which permits the operator to cut, dissolve, or wipe between the selected views. The chosen image is relayed to the recorder where the final picture is viewed on the production monitor.

Sound

The soundtrack is as important as the picture in a video recording and should be accorded just as much care and attention in achieving quality and choosing equipment.

Microphones having different characteristics are chosen to suit a specific task. Omnidirectional microphones accept sound from all directions; cardioid accept sound in a broad beam from one direction and unidirectional in a narrow beam; bidirectional microphones operate like a pair of cardioids back to back, and so on. Generally speaking, and where feasible, each sound source should be microphoned or monitored separately and sound fed back to the video recorder through a sound mixing unit on which the individual volume levels can be adjusted and controlled. Assessing the quality and level of sound should always be done through earphones plugged into the recorder where, in terms of the recording, true values can be judged. Microphones need to be positioned so that they cause the least intrusion into the picture and this can be achieved, for example, by slinging them on poles, or by using tiny lapel or tie clip units for individual participants.

Lighting

The quantity and quality of light affects the quality of the picture in a number of ways. Poor light lowers the brilliance of the picture, it dulls and alters the colours, and, most importantly, it reduces the depth of field—that is, the distance between the nearest and most distant points at which all subjects can be brought into sharp focus. Having sufficient light on the scene, or using a camera of very high sensitivity, is vital for obtaining sharp, brilliant pictures.

Lighting arrangement is a skill requiring practice and experiment and it is worth spending time on it. Professionals often use the basic three point method which uses a key, a fill, and a back light. The key light should be the brightest as it provides most of the illumination and should be placed in front of the subject, slightly to one side (usually the left) and fairly high (20–45 degrees). As by itself the key light tends to create hard shadows on the subject, a less intense light placed on the opposite side will fill these dark areas. Finally, another light, again softer than the key, is directed towards the back of the subject and from above (so called rim lighting) in order to make the subject stand out and separate it from the background.

Editing

Editing is the process by which a video programme is compiled. It includes the removal of unwanted material and the assembling of various shots, titles, graphics, etc, in their correct sequence. With cinematograph film this task is relatively simple as it is done by physically cutting up the film and joining the selected pieces together with film cement. It is also precise because each complete picture, representing one twenty fourth of a second of action, is visible on the film. With video recording the invisible electronic picture signals are laid down in a diagonal pattern on the tape and unless this pattern of lines can be precisely maintained when editing from one shot to another the subsequent picture disintegrates. Video tape editing is therefore an electronic process and entails the use of two linked recorders; one, the master, on which all the prerecorded material is played; the other, the slave—which must have an inbuilt edit facility—on which the selected material is compiled and recorded in sequence. Editing equipment can be as simple as this, and somewhat imprecise, or it can be highly complex and accurate with the ability to accept inputs from video recordings, cameras, film, sound recordings, microphones, etc; able to fade, dissolve, and superimpose images; and with an electronic controller that permits the editor to rehearse the edits and make cuts at precise points.

Planning

Today's technology has made video production deceptively simple; so simple in fact that there is a tendency to ignore the most important task in creating an effective videotape—planning. Even the most basic production needs planning and some form of rehearsal if disaster is to be avoided. For example, at a point in the recording of a clinical consultation the cameraman is concentrating on a close up view of the patient's face while he describes his symptoms. Through the viewfinder the patient's face is all that the cameraman can see. Then, without any verbal cue, the doctor begins to examine the patient's hands, while the patient continues his verbal report. Seconds later the cameraman realises that the point of interest has changed and makes a desperate attempt to retrain and refocus his camera, by which time the doctor has turned his attention to the patient's eyes. The action, perhaps very important to the story, has been lost and the camera chase continues. Preplanning and rehearsal of the action, camera position and angles, etc, is therefore vital even in a simple, unscripted, one man, unedited production.

More complex productions require much greater and more precise planning, and a storyboard is essential especially if editing is to be done. A proper storyboard or production script will consist of the following information, usually laid out in columns with across the page reference. The "sequence," which is identified by a number, relates to a particular portion of the script and this may be broken down into a number of different preplanned "shots" each having its own identifying number. Any shot may require several attempts or "takes" to get it right and the usable one is identified by number and its position on the tape is noted from the tape counter number on the recorder. "Pix" are brief descriptions and camera instructions for the picture elements in each shot, for example, "zoom in to CU (close up) of patient's face, tilt down to CU of hands, tilt up to CU of patient's eyes, pull back to reveal doctor and patient." The "sound" column includes the script of the actual words to be spoken and identifies the live elements recorded on the spot and "voice over" (VO) or narration which is added on afterwards. The "FX" columns—and there may be several—contain details of any sound effects (background noise, etc) and where they fade in, up, down, or out. Finally, the music; this is identified separately and in detail and usually added at the editing stage.

This may seem over elaborate but without a detailed plan known by everyone concerned on the production, chaos will inevitably ensue, time be wasted, and tempers fray.

Legal responsibilities

It is important to understand that in compiling a video pro-gramme the use of any copyright material, whether it be a diagram from a textbook, a film extract, a still photograph, or a piece of music (live or recorded), is unlawful without the express per-mission of the copyright owner.

The Video Recording Act 1984 and the Child Protection Act 1978 place restrictions on the recording of certain subjects, and on the distribution and showing of video recordings that contain material which under the acts is considered to be indecent or displaying gross violence. Producers and users of medical and scientific video recordings are advised to take extreme care in this matter and they may well be surprised by the nature of material classified under these headings. Equally important in medical recordings is the matter of confidentiality of illustrative clinical recordings of patients, and both these subjects are covered in the North East Thames Regional Health Authority's code of practice listed below.

Useful reading

Owen D, Dunton M. *The complete handbook of video.* Harmondsworth: Penguin, 1982.

Watts H. *On camera: how to produce film and video.* London: BBC Publications, 1982.

Basic video guide (£1) and *Code of practice on the confidentiality of illustrative clinical records* (£5). North East Thames Regional Health Authority Audio Visual Advisory Committee, Robin Brook Centre, St Bartholomew's Hospital, West Smithfield, London EC1A 7BE.

Devise a course for overseas visitors who don't speak English well

B B SEEDHOM, J E SMEATHERS, D T THOMPSON

Running a residential course requires thorough planning. This is particularly so when the delegates are from a country where the first language is not English. A group from the rheumatism research unit in Leeds recently ran such a course. The subject was biomechanics, particularly of the knee, and the audience was a group of orthopaedic surgeons from Japan who visited this country for 12 days. The need for such a course had been firmly identified, and it was seen as an opportunity to form links between us and the medical profession in Japan while raising funds for the unit. This chapter describes the problems we found, the strategies we adopted, and our successes (and failures) in presenting this particular course.

Aims of the course

Persuading a group of professionals to devote considerable time and money to a course requires that a definite need for the course has been established. In our case this was identified in a paper describing the state of biomechanical research in orthopaedics in Japan.[1] The paper was based on a questionnaire sent to medical schools in Japan with orthopaedic departments. One of the conclusions was that "the majority of (Japanese) orthopaedists involved in bioengineering research feel the lack of engineering knowledge and technique and have a desire to gain such knowledge." We decided that a short, intensive bioengineering course on a subject of mutual interest would be attractive to Japanese surgeons.

The aims of the course must be made clear, and all organisers must be aware of them. It is best to start with organisational aims—namely, why and how you intend to run the course—and work down to the specific educational aims. These should be written down and circulated for discussion. Some members of the team may well disagree with the aims. If this cannot be overcome by discussion they may decide not to contribute. This can be disappointing, but it is far better to find out at this stage than to produce, after days of preparation, material that is inconsistent.

The aims of the bioengineering course were split into two groups. The organisational aims were: to form links with the orthopaedic profession in Japan; to raise funds for the research unit; and to provide an attractive package comprising both technical education and recreation. The educational aims were: to ensure that the participants left with a working knowledge of the fundamentals of engineering mechanics and materials science on which orthopaedic biomechanics is based; to provide an insight into the way engineers in general, and bioengineers in particular, approach a problem; to provide a series of lectures on a particular topic of bioengineering to illustrate this; and to make the surgeons aware of the work in progress in the major centres of bioengineering in Great Britain.

Anticipated problems and preparation

When delegates commit themselves to the expense of time away from work, and possibly a long overseas journey, the organisers are under a heavy obligation to provide a professional service. Most of this is to do with attention to detail: clearly presented lectures, well maintained and tested equipment, comfortable lecture theatres, adequate meals and accommodation, and efficient transport. None of these is appreciably different from the problems encountered in organising any residential course. It is important, however, to try to predict problems specific to the particular course and audience, especially any problems related to language.

All the surgeons on our course could read and write English. Most, however, were not used to assimilating spoken English. Our previous experience with Japanese visitors to the unit had made us aware that the normal type of lecture presentation would not be adequate. The problems of communicating with an audience in a language other than their own were exacerbated in this case by the need for specialist terminology. Much of this—for example, the terms "stress" and "strain"—causes particular problems owing to the confusion of meaning between uses in the engineering and medical professions.

As far as the engineering course was concerned, it was not easy to predict how familiar the participants would be with the concepts of engineering mechanics. It was, therefore, difficult to decide at what level it would be appropriate to start this part of the course. It is our experience that mechanical concepts are really appreciated only when they are applied in solving problems. Without a grasp of these concepts the students would be unable to appreciate fully the specialist lectures in the course. We were concerned, however, about the reaction of a group of surgeons to an "examples class" approach, where they would be asked to make calculations and answer questions reinforcing the main points of the previous lecture.

Many of the group would be visiting Britain for the first time. Although they were anxious to make the most of their visit academically, it was clear that filling their available time with lectures alone would be counterproductive. Ideally they should be able to recover after their journey, be given time to accustom themselves to the language before facing serious academic tasks, and know that there would be adequate time for sightseeing and shopping.

Discussions about the aims and design of the package deal took place roughly one year before the event. From the start one of the organisers was a surgeon in Japan who looked at our ideas, discussed them with colleagues, and made suggestions. In doing this he also acted as our local advertising agent by bringing the course to the attention of possible delegates.

In consultation with our Japanese colleagues we decided that the right mixture of recreation and education would be achieved with a 14 day package deal. Air travel to and from Tokyo would occupy one day each way, which would allow 12 days in Britain. Most of the academic material would be presented as a three day intensive course. We decided that the best way of providing an appreciation of current bioengineering research was for the surgeons to visit various well known centres. The time before and after the course would, therefore, include visits to such centres, as well as providing time for recovery, acclimatisation to the new language, sightseeing, and shopping.

As the package began to take shape it became clear that we needed someone to take responsibility for the travel and accommodation. Consequently we appointed a secretary for the equivalent of one day a week for the four months before the event. She was taken on full time during the two week visit. As the Japanese party signed up for the trip they arranged for a tour guide who could speak English to liaise with us. This guide eventually travelled to Britain with the party and proved invaluable. With hindsight we would strongly recommend this arrangement of secretary and tour guide taking joint responsibility for the organisation of the trip, while a member of the visiting party should be available to advise on the academic aspects of the course.

The size of the party was finalised a month before the event. The detailed itinerary had to be decided on at this stage so that hotel bookings could be made taking advantage of discounts for large parties and early bookings (table). Hotels were booked close to the bioengineering centres and sightseeing areas that the party wished to visit. The university conference centre at Leeds was booked for the short period of the course. No special meals were requested by the delegates, so traditional English fare was provided throughout their stay. Our visitors did, however, make regular use of local Chinese restaurants.

Itinerary of fortnight's course on biomechanical engineering for Japanese orthopaedic surgeons

Day	Day of week	Time	Activity
1	Thursday		Air travel from Tokyo
2	Friday	0605	Arrive Heathrow from Hong Kong; breakfast at Strand Palace Hotel
		1100	Imperial College Bioengineering Centre
3	Saturday		At leisure in London; overnight stay at Strand Palace Hotel
4	Sunday		Journey to Leeds via Cambridge; accommodation at university conference centre
5	Monday		Sightseeing in Yorkshire, Harrogate, Fountains Abbey, and Ripon
6	Tuesday ⎫		
7	Wednesday ⎬		Three day course
8	Thursday ⎭		
		1700	Conference dinner at Ripon
9	Friday		Journey to Edinburgh via Alnwick, Bamburgh castle, and Lindisfarne
10	Saturday		At leisure in Edinburgh
11	Sunday		Journey to Chester via Moffat and Windermere
12	Monday		Journey to Oxford via Stratford on Avon
13	Tuesday	0900	Nuffield Orthopaedic Engineering Centre, Oxford
		1530	Depart for London; overnight stay at Excelsior Hotel, Heathrow
14	Wednesday	0915	Air travel to Tokyo

A luxury coach, which was available for the entire period of the package, was used for transport. Although there were periods when the coach was idle, it had many advantages over alternatives such as trains, hired cars, and local buses. It provided an economical and flexible door to door service and so allowed the maximum use of available time with little risk of losing people in transit. The tour guide was able to ensure that overall schedules were maintained while the visitors themselves had considerable control over what they did and saw within that schedule.

Course details

During the planning of the three day course of lectures it became apparent that the greatest problem of communication was that the students were unfamiliar with spoken English. To assess the magnitude of this problem we performed a full dress rehearsal of the course before the delegates arrived. All the lecturers and demonstrators on the course were present while each lecturer presented his lecture in full. Fortunately, two of the lecturers—an engineer researching into a related subject and an orthopaedic surgeon, both working in the university—were Japanese and thus able to offer helpful comments. Each lecture was evaluated on the basis of content, level of understanding required, structure, clarity of presentation, how the various aids were to be used (slides, models, and visual aids), and, most importantly, the language. All idiomatic phrases (well; I am afraid; it is all very well but, etc) had to be omitted. Complex phrases were made much simpler, and a consistent and limited vocabulary was adhered to. Jargon and technical terms were explained as they occurred, and emphasis was placed on diction. It is not easy for a foreigner to understand garbled pronunciation, especially when two or more words have the same sound but completely different meanings. The speed of delivery was also slowed down to that which our Japanese lecturers could follow. We found it helpful if one of the organisers sat at the back of the lecture room as a monitor. His function was to alert the speaker if he spoke too fast or too quietly. The dress rehearsal also enabled us to check the seating arrangements in the lecture theatre and the audiovisual equipment. We considered that uniformity of the seating arrangements was essential. Although this would appear to be an obvious aspect of organising any course, it is seldom paid enough attention. Often there are first and second

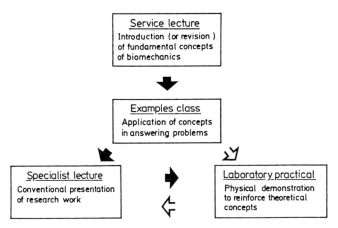

Generalised strategy of lecture presentation showing how each specialist lecture was supported by extra lectures and preparation work.

class seats: an overhead projector may obscure vision, or its noisy cooling fan may reduce audibility. To avoid these problems each seat was examined individually for clarity of sight and sound. Projectors were placed as far back as possible to reduce the noise (this of course would not be a problem in a purpose built auditorium with a back projection room).

In addition to the slow delivery we decided that a visual display of the key words of each lecture was required. To avoid loss of continuity of the theme of the lecture two slide projectors and screens were used. One screen carried the theme slides while the other carried the key words relevant to the slide. A booklet was provided that included the same list of key words so that the student could find the correct page at any time by comparing the listed key words with those on the screen. The booklet contained space for the student to take notes about each concept. Other audiovisual materials were used only when absolutely necessary—for instance, overhead projectors were used for graphs, and previously prepared diagrams and working models were used to provide tangible evidence of the concepts being discussed. Video tapes were also used to show points of interest and concepts that could not be readily shown in the lecture room.

The core of the course was a series of specialist lectures about biomechanical aspects of the human knee joint, its kinematic function, loading and force transmission, commonly occurring damage, and techniques of surgical repair and prosthetic replacement of the knee. To appreciate this material fully a working knowledge of the concepts of bioengineering was required. We also needed to ensure that the audience had a common level of understanding of these concepts. The specialist lectures on the knee were, therefore, interwoven with a series of "service lectures" that provided this theoretical background. The theory was made relevant by closely tailoring each service lecture to the needs of the following specialist lecture. Similarly, the topics of the specialist lectures were presented in such a sequence that the teaching of engineering concepts could be developed in a structured way. At crucial points in the development of the theory the lectures were supplemented with examples classes. These were designed both to give the students the opportunity to exercise the analytical tools that they were being introduced to and to allow us to monitor the progress of the students to ensure that the lectures were being presented at the appropriate level. The figure shows the hierarchy of the various types of lectures used during the course.

Appraisal of the course

It is instructive and valuable to know for future reference how successful the course was through discussion with all those who participated. A good structure for this is to work through original aims and assess how successful the course was in achieving each goal. It is also useful if each participant makes a written list of what he considers were the successes and failures. A questionnaire given to the audience before they leave may be helpful. If this is to be of value it must be well thought out and the time required to prepare it not underestimated.[2] It must be prepared in advance of the course and be ready for the audience immediately the course ends.

We drew several conclusions about our course from discussions with the delegates. The course was very favourably received. Many delegates admitted that they had had low expectations of how much they would be able to learn owing to the communication problem but that they had been pleasantly surprised. The rehearsal of all the service lectures and most of the specialist lectures ensured the smooth running and continuity of the lecture course, the benefits of which were so apparent that we would recommend that this should form an important part of any lecture course. The use of key words on the second projector screen was certainly worth the extra éffort required in the presentation. The examples classes were surprisingly successful in that the delegates enjoyed them and often completed them before the end of the session. This may have been helped by the intensely competitive temperament within this particular group. Others benefited from the one to one discussion that was possible because of the number of staff available during examples classes.

The prepared notebook was not as well used as had been hoped. It is easy to underestimate the skill required in taking lecture notes, especially when this problem is compounded by the use of a second language. The notebooks did, however, serve as a useful aide memoire for the delegates to take home with them at the end of the course. Many of the delegates used cameras in the lecture theatre, and some even had miniature tape recorders. Perhaps this easily available technology could be used to reduce the need for taking notes on future courses.

The excursions to places of historical interest were much enjoyed, and the ratio of one academic to two recreational days proved to be an acceptable balance. The tour guide was useful as he was able to advise us about the major subjects of interest within the touring party, and this resulted in an impromptu trip to St Andrews golf course. In retrospect we could have tailored the recreation more closely to the interests of our party if we had contacted the tour guide before their arrival. We certainly underestimated the Japanese interest in golf.

1   Terajama K. The present state of biomechanical research in orthopaedics in Japan—an observation by an orthopaedic surgeon. *Eng Med* 1983; **12**: 207–9.
2   Youngman M B. *Designing and analysing questionnaires*. Nottingham: University of Nottingham, 1978. (Rediguide 12.)

Signpost your hospital

J H BARON

Those who work in institutions know where they are and where they are going; they are rarely conscious of the notices and sign-posts. Doctors should, but alas do not, have more awareness of the problem of patients and visitors all of whom, quite apart from their specific diagnostic fears, are frightened of the health care system in general and of hospitals in particular.

Patients and visitors have to make their way to a hospital and can be helped by a map being included in the literature sent out before admission. They need signs to tell them that they have arrived. They need to reach a particular part of the hospital and to know when they have achieved this objective. Each sign must be pre-cisely located, of suitable size, material, and colour, and made up of legible and beautiful letters that suit the building.[1]

Anyone concerned with signposting a hospital must obtain a copy of the Department of Health and Social Security's *Signs*[2] which provides full details of the Health Signs system and language. This chapter offers a personal user's guide for those who care about the visual environment of their hospital, whether old[3] or new,[4] and want to try to make their hospital both more efficient and more attractive.

Practicalities

The planner should pretend that he or she is, in turn, a driver, passenger, or pedestrian coming to the hospital, who needs to park, to reach a specific department, and from there other departments, and then to be able to find the lavatories, the cafeteria, and then the way out and back to the car park, all the necessary signs being still visible at dusk and by night.

Signs to the hospital

Those arriving at rail, underground, or bus stations need clear signs pointing towards the hospital, as from London Bridge station to Guy's. Those foolish enough to go to Hammersmith underground station hoping to find themselves near the Hammersmith Hospital may need a kindly notice referring them to White City or East Acton stations instead. Car drivers need clear signs from town centres or major roads to the correct turn offs. Many older hospitals are in back streets and they need signs from the nearest main road.

Proclaiming the hospital

Some public buildings can be arrogantly anonymous, like London clubs or Oxford and Cambridge colleges. A hospital should proclaim its name, be proud of its identity and its work, and assure visitors that they have come to the correct building.

Such declamation was taken for granted by the voluntary hospitals of the nineteenth century; the workhouse infirmaries skulked in shameful anonymity. There are still good Georgian examples in London such as St George's, Hyde Park Corner (designed by Wilkin, 1827) and the General Lying-in Hospital, York Road, (Harris, 1828). No one can mistake the Royal Waterloo Hospital for Children and Women (Nicholson, 1903–5) with its giant raised lettering in Doulton tiles.

The tradition continued into the 1930s in a variety of media. Westminster Hospital (Pearson, 1937) has raised metal letters on the façade to Horseferry Road, cut out metal letters lit internally at night over the main entrance, and letters incised in stone on the nurses' home. About that time came enamel on metal for smaller signs (for example, the Gordon Hospital). When the workhouse infirmary in Du Cane Road graduated into a teaching institution an elegant sign of metal letters on stone arose and can still be seen between the gates: HAMMERSMITH HOSPITAL AND P.ST GRADUATE SCHOOL.. LONDON—having lost a few letters over the years.

The new Royal Free Hospital has preserved its 1894 semicircular cast iron sign from the old building, used classical raised metal letters for its school of medicine's façade, and used bold capitals mounted on a strip away from the main entrance wall to the new hospital. Neurologists (Maida Vale Hospital; Institute of Neurology) and psychiatrists (Tavistock Centre) stick to large plain capitals. But then came Health Service lettering (see below).

Finding the part that you want

Taxi drivers and some motorists need clear directions about where to drop passengers—be they patients or visitors—depending on whether they want accident and emergency, outpatients, or the main entrance for visitors. If departments are in independent buildings it is even more important that outpatients, obstetrics, physiotherapy, etc be signposted from the main road to the car parks nearest these units.

Car park notices, like all hospital notices, should not convey simply the usual warnings (CONSULTANTS ONLY), threats (YOUR WHEELS WILL BE CLAMPED), menaces (PENALTY £20), and disclaimers (BOARD OF GOVERNORS NOT RESPONSIBLE FOR LOSSES). Notices should be courteous and helpful: WELCOME TO ST CECILIA'S: PLEASE PARK HERE.

From the car park clear signs for the main entrance and inquiries should be placed so that no one, however anxious, could either fail to proceed in the desired direction or be left in limbo at an unmarked crossroads with alternative paths. Remember that many of your visitors have never been to your hospital before: do help them. Do not be tempted into the false economy of a small monochrome map surrounded and financed by local advertisements. Try for large maps showing, from the visitor's point of view and position ("You are here"), which buildings have which wards and departments on which floor, and by which staircase and lift they can be reached, with appropriate colour coding of the areas of different use. Designers specialising in axonometric drawings can construct these plans so that they differ only from the viewpoint of direction of approach. The alternatives are mere banks of signs which can confuse by multiplicity, unless they are grouped and broken down in the stages: ALL WARDS/OUTPATIENTS/ACCIDENT & EMERGENCY as the visitor approaches a particular group. Try to be consistent: different signs in succession, such as ACCIDENT & EMERGENCY/CASUALTY/EMERGENCIES, but all going to the same department are disorientating to the hapless patient.

Nor should the main entrance be negativistic. Visitors are not charmed by their first impression of an NHS hospital—NO SMOKING/SILENCE/NO CHILDREN UNDER 14. Why not WELCOME TO ST

CECILIA'S, A NO SMOKING HOSPITAL and PLEASE HELP US TO HELP OUR PATIENTS BY TALKING QUIETLY?

Signs for wards and departments and lifts

Although some of the older workhouse infirmaries still have wards signified by letters and numbers, most hospitals new and old have wards identified by a name, usually of a person, but occasionally of a saint, street, or electoral ward. A personal touch is given to a ward name if it is accompanied by a photograph or print of that person together with a brief biographical note. The Royal Free Hospital has a particularly successful set. Departments can be handled similarly and named after former directors.

Elevators need detailed lists—both beside each lift button on each floor and inside the lift—of the wards and departments on each level. It is helpful if when the lift stops at each floor passengers see through the open gates a giant number on the wall opposite denoting the level, and similarly for those climbing stairs. As you arrive on a floor you need signs for the direction and location of each unit on that floor. Directions can be in identical format on each level, but it is then helpful to have the floor you are at picked out in a special colour.

Other signs

The tendency now is to number all doors. These also should have a name, indicating the room's function or occupant, and the hospital needs some central, identifiable, responsible, and dynamic person who can order such name boards and indeed all other signs. Nothing is worse than handwritten scraps of paper taped on to doors, windows, or walls. Of course, temporary notes are needed; they should be put neatly on prominent blank noticeboards. More formal events boards with movable letters should list the timetable of the day or week.

Maintenance

If your signs are washable or polishable then someone must wash and polish them regularly; if they are painted they will need painting often, and if they are separate letters fixed to a wall they may go askew or fall off.

Battle of the styles—which lettering?

The NHS has a typeface—Health Alphabet—all of its own (fig 1). It is widely assumed by health service architects, designers, and administrators, and even by doctors, that the DHSS requires all hospitals to use this alphabet and no other when using the Health Signs language. This is a total misconception. The DHSS indeed prefers hospitals to use Health Alphabet for economy, legibility and a recognisable style, but *Signs* recognises individualism, and gives examples in Garamond, Clarendon, and Rockwell. *Signs* rightly points out that, whatever style of lettering is chosen, there should be consistency of type for all the signs in a particular building and with the authority's coat of arms, symbol, and logo.

The early hospitals had lettering chosen presumably by their architects to be consistent with the style of the building. St George's is neoclassical, and the raised gilt lettering on the architrave of the portico is in a suitable neoclassical style, a formal announcement of classical monumentality in serifed letters. Most hospitals for the next 100 years retained a classical letter form. The alternative, a Roman letter without serifs, appeared on the Brighton Pavilion (1784), as English Egyptian type (1816), and Grotesque ("Grot") in 1835.[5] With the beginning of the modern movement in architecture, design, and typography, the sans serif letter form was revived and has been widely used in the past 70 years, especially in Germany since the Bauhaus.

In 1915 Edward Johnston was commissioned by Frank Pick of London Transport to design the first standardised lettering for systematic use by a large organisation. The sans serif London Underground typeface has survived successfully to this day. Johnston's pupil, Eric Gill, produced a sans serif type design of Sans in 1927, which has developed into a family of different weights and widths. The medical world soon followed the trend, for example, in the London School of Hygiene and Tropical Medicine built in 1928 (Horder and Rees).[1]

The aesthetic problem of public lettering became acute when the Ministry of Transport's departmental committee on traffic signs reported in 1944, "that as legibility is important the standard lettering which we use for traffic signs is suitable for street names."[6] Local authorities were recommended to use a standard sans serif. Only rearguard action by letter lovers and the Royal Fine Art Commission persuaded the ministry to include in the

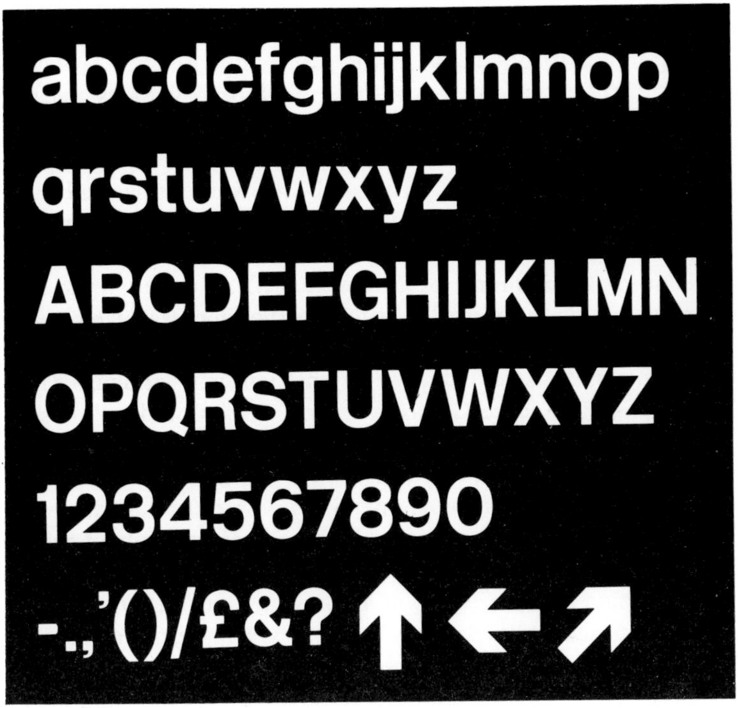

abcdefghijklmnop
qrstuvwxyz
ABCDEFGHIJKLMN
OPQRSTUVWXYZ
1234567890
-.,'()/£&? ↑ ← ↗

Fig 1—Health Alphabet.

recommended designs a serif alphabet, specially designed by David Kindersley in 1947.[6] When motorway lettering was to be standardised, however, Sir Colin Anderson's committee chose on aesthetic grounds Jock Kinneir's monoline sans serif upper and lower case (originally designed for the P & O and Orient lines, and later adapted for London Airport), rather than the Kindersley all capital serif, in spite of the latter's being shown by the Road Research Laboratory to be more legible, even though the difference was not statistically significant.

Sans serif letters then strengthened their hold. In 1957 Max Miedinger had redesigned a Basle typefounder's Grotesque. Renamed Helvetica it has had since the early 1960s almost universal success, not only as a typeface for printers, but also for signs particularly since it became available as "Letrasign." In the late 1960s the DHSS commissioned Jock Kinneir to produce Health Alphabet, which is between a Helvetica light and Helvetica medium.[2] Health Alphabet, often called NHS lettering, has

119

engulfed our hospitals old and new, just as when BEA and BOAC merged into British Airways in 1973 they chose for their new corporate identity a sans serif so as to seem informal, friendly, caring, and non-pompous to the new young traveller.[6] Unfortunately, as Kinneir's Health Alphabet, Railway Alphabet and Airport Alphabet (designed by Fletcher, Forbes and Crosby) are so similar, their separate identities are lost. It is interesting that Colin Banks and John Miles gave the Post Office a totally different style of lettering in yellow on a red ground for its new image.[7]

Adrian Frutiger designed the signs for the Charles de Gaulle airport in Paris: his Roissy is a thin, elegant sans serif reminiscent of the Johnston Sans of 1915. When the new and fabulous MacKenzie Health Science Centre was built in Edmonton, Professor Bartl was asked to direct a project to design a sign system.[8] Their studies on legibility led him to Frutiger 55 Roman (fig 2), which was therefore chosen throughout to "combine the advantages of modern sans-serif faces with the elegance and sensibility of classic type design."

But fashion in lettering, as in architecture and design, has now turned back again to the classical. Anthony Williams, consultant in signposting to the DHSS, has at St Bartholomew's Hospital used different alphabets (including a traditional serif type, Garamond), which are related in terms of colour, size, and proportion to the design of buildings of different periods. In 1983 I persuaded St Charles's Hospital to use Times New Roman (fig 3) throughout its 1881 buildings, and this lettering was also chosen for the new mental health buildings of 1985. Times New Roman was of course designed as a typeface for close viewing, with marked difference between thick and thin strokes, and is therefore not suitable for large buildings where notices are seen from afar. Both the British Museum and the National Gallery have recently redesigned all their signs, notices, and labels using letters with serifs: their designers, independently, and quite unknown to each other, chose Century Bold and Old, classical and monumental serifed typefaces (fig 4).

Doctors and scientists reading this account should by now be thinking of James Lind, and demand a controlled trial of legibility. Unfortunately, there have been few such studies in relation to signs, and the results conflict. When the laboratory evidence favoured serif, a committee still chose a sans serif upper and lower case for the motorway (see above). Several studies have rejected

Occupational
Therapy

External Psychiatric
Services

Provincial Laboratory

Exit 114 Street

Cafeteria

Information Desk

X-Ray

Occupational
Therapy

Emergency

Fig 2—Sample settings of Frutiger 55 Roman.

Times New Roman

ABCDEFGHIJKLMNOPQRSTUVWXYZ
abcdefghijklmnopqrstuvwxyz
123456789 ()!,.?;"

Fig 3—Times New Roman.

Century Bold

ABCDEFGHIJKLMNOPQRSTUVWXYZ
abcdefghijklmnopqrstuvwxyz
123456789 ()!,.?;"

Fig 4—Century Bold.

Helvetica and their related typefaces because they do not differentiate enough between individual letter forms to give optimum legibility of signs.

Other languages

Hospital managers automatically assume that notices should be in the English language in Latin script. Many parts of Britain have in their catchment areas ethnic groups with languages with non-Latin scripts—for example, Greek and Bengali. Expert advice should be taken to produce signs as beautiful and as legible as possible in these typefaces.

Conclusion

New hospitals must have a complete sign system, and most old hospitals will benefit from a revamping of the miscellaneous notices that have grown up over the decades. Remember, the system of signs is codified[2]; what you must decide is the type of letter. Basically, in the absence of good scientific field trials of legibility of signs, including their suitability for people with impaired vision, choices are still made on personal aesthetic grounds.

Certainly, use NHS lettering if you want to avoid controversy and save time, if you think it is the most beautiful available, and if you want your hospital to look like every other institution. If you want a modern sans serif, then there are several that are both legible and beautiful. If you prefer serifed letters then you should look at old and new buildings that have them, until you find one you like which will suit your building. Then decide whether you want capitals or small letters. The choices are yours. Seize your opportunities—provided you are confident that you will not be upset by the inevitable criticism of your decisions.

I am grateful for helpful discussions or correspondence with Professor Peter Bartl (Edmonton), Peter Dormer (Ealing), Professor Fred Halter (Berne), Tony Noakes (DHSS), Professor Michael Twyman (Reading), John Weeks (London), Anthony Williams (Harpenden), Iden Wickings (London). None of them is responsible for any of my opinions, errors, or conclusions.

1 Bartram A. *Lettering in architecture*. London: Lund Humphries, 1975.
2 Williams A, ed. *Signs*. DHSS Health Technical Memorandum 65. London: HMSO, 1984.
3 Baron J H. How to beautify your old hospital. *Br Med J* 1984; **239:** 807–10.
4 Baron J H, Greene L. *Art in hospitals. Funding works of art in new hospitals. Murals in London hospitals. Br Med J* 1984; **289:** 1731–7.
5 McLean R. *The Thames and Hudson manual of typography*. London: Thames and Hudson, 1980.
6 Crutchley B. *To be a printer*. London: Bodley Head, 1980.
7 Dormer P. *A closer look: lettering* London: Crafts Council, 1983.
8 Bartl P. *Some pitfalls in signage systems for hospitals*. Icographic I/II Denmark: Mobilia Press, 1982.

Represent your colleagues

JAMES APPLEYARD

Doctors' prime interest is the care of their patients. As this is sufficiently time consuming and professionally rewarding it is not surprising that relatively few doctors become interested in representing their colleagues. Clinical work entails looking after individuals rather than groups, and doctors have traditionally worked independently rather than collectively. When conflicts between the profession and government arise efforts are made to get the profession to act collectively. Yet we must always remember that it is this individuality and independence that are the centre of our professional power. Like all power, if it is too tightly centralised it is much easier to take over and destroy.

It takes some gross intrusion into our professional freedom, such as the action by Barbara Castle in 1975 over private practice, and more recently by Norman Fowler with the implementation of the "limited list" to galvanise groups of doctors into collective protest and action. Most doctors have a deep sense of justice and fairness that is inherent in their everyday practice. Over the years they have tolerated a slow but inexorable erosion of their pay and status, and only when the pace of change is precipitate or acts of gross unfairness are inflicted upon them do they raise sufficient voices in unison. Other perennial issues, such as "manpower" rightly interest young doctors in particular as their future careers are at stake. At these times the majority will look to the minority of doctors who represent them for action, and many of those seeking action will themselves get involved in the medicopolitical process. Few doctors have set out on a medicopolitical career for its own sake. The issues are interesting—often far reaching—and competition is challenging, but the rewards fall far short of those achieved through clinical practice in relation to the enormous amount of work that is generated. There are, however, those who do so primarily to achieve wider political ends. They can be sustained by a small minority of support on narrow issues, but the need to reflect the broad view of the profession, the hard work required, and the democratic accountability of the main medicopolitical forum, the British Medical Association (BMA), has militated against "party" political domination of medical affairs. Impatience, intolerance, and frustration with this democratic process breed pressure groups, who wax and wane according to the issues of the time unless they are propped up by wider political interests. Pressure groups have proved good training grounds for medical politicians. They command a disproportionate amount of power in relation to their numbers by the interest generated in the media. They make good copy in challenging the establishment and because of the relatively small numbers, they are able to work as a closely knit team with limited but usually well defined objectives. Challenging authority is one of the quickest ways of learning how the system works even if the system is thereby turned against you. Pressure groups rarely have the resources either in members or money to cover a great variety of medical, political, and professional activities and interests. They rapidly find that they cannot impose their views on the reluctant majority as there are limits at any particular time as to what the profession will wear. Inevitably, to survive, the pressure group has to parasitise on the larger organisation with greater resources and access to better information. It takes time to change attitudes and often in this process, which requires a lot of patience, members of the pressure group get absorbed into the wider stream of BMA politics and adjust to these wider loyalties.

Knowledge of his fellow doctors, knowledge of the current medicopolitical issues, and knowledge of the system are the three pillars on which an effective representative must stand. How effective he or she is depends on flair, ability, timing, and luck. There are also some skills that should be acquired.

The system

Exciting scientific and technological advances have made rapid changes in medicine and in the public's expectation of what medicine in general and doctors in particular should achieve. Progess in communication has made possible the widest dissemination of medical information, and patients rightly expect more time from doctors to discuss their problems and help them make their own decisions. In contrast the state system has tended to impede this process by making medicine more impersonal.

Doctors traditionally worked as independent professionals whose main source of income was their patients. Third parties appeared when insurance schemes were introduced, and with the inception of the NHS in 1948 the medical scene was dominated by the government as the near monopoly employer of doctors. General practitioners have fortunately retained some of their independence as they are independent contractors, but hospital and community health service doctors, who need more expensive support services, have essentially become full time employees. The interests of the two groups may conflict at times and there have been repeated attempts to encourage a full time salaried service for all doctors. The present arrangements, however, together with the freedom that consultants have to practise independently of the health service, have probably been the main reasons why doctors have retained a considerable amount of independence in their work.

The General Medical Council

The interrelationship of the government, the DHSS, the NHS as the employer, and the profession as employees is complex. On the profession's side, power is shared. No one body represents all doctors' interests. The General Medical Council (GMC) has been given statutory powers to allow the profession a considerable amount of self regulation. It is responsible for maintaining the standards of medical practice and for coordinating all stages of medical education, both undergraduate and postgraduate. Though half of the GMC is now elected, the traditional domination of the council by university academics continues. With only a small proportion of the profession voting and with a large number of candidates interested in gaining a place on the council, the elections have proved an ideal hunting ground for minority groups. The BMA, on whose initiative the GMC was founded, has gained more influence recently.

Colleges and committees

The royal colleges are responsible for the standards of practice in their own specialties and have become increasingly responsive to the views of their fellows and members. They are consulted directly by ministers and the DHSS. Their peripheral influence lies in their activities on advisory appointments committees for new consultants and in their recognition of training posts in the health service. They are not directly concerned with the terms and conditions of doctors but have joined with the BMA and their senior and junior hospital doctor representatives to form the Joint Consultants Committee. This negotiates agreements with the DHSS through meetings with the Chief Medical Officer on professional matters. This is an important meeting ground as far as hospital doctors are concerned for it brings the professional side, the royal colleges, and the political side, the BMA, together. A parallel structure exists for community medicine whereby the Faculty of Community Medicine and the Central Committee for Community Medicine and Community Health meet the Deputy Chief Medical Officer in the form of the Community Medicine Consultative Committee.

The political wing of the profession is the BMA. It became a trade union under the Trades Union and Labour Relations Act of 1974. It is not affiliated to the Trades Union Council though it has retained links with the TUC over many years. The BMA is recognised by the health departments and local health authorities as the negotiating body. Ministers and health authorities may talk to other groups but no agreements binding on the profession can be made. The BMA is a recognised staff organisation representing the medical profession on the General Whitley Council, which on the staff side is composed of several unions, including the National Union of Public Employees, the Confederation of Hospital Service Employees, the BMA, the Royal College of Nursing, and Royal College of Midwives. In this forum terms and conditions of service for all NHS staff, including doctors, are negotiated. By special arrangement, the hospital and dental services are covered by the agreements reached in the General Whitley Council only if representatives of the BMA's senior doctors (the Central Committee for Hospital Medical Services), junior doctors (the Hospital Junior Staffs Committee), and community staff (the Central Committee for Community Medicine and Community Health) jointly agree that they should be. The hospital senior and junior staff join together in a joint negotiating committee with the DHSS, and the community physicians and community health staff have a separate negotiating board. The level of pay—as opposed to the detailed discussions on terms and conditions of service—is determined by the government on the recommendation of the independent review body. Evidence to this body is given each year by representatives of the negotiating teams of all the major craft committees of the BMA. General practitioners are independent contractors to the family practitioner committees. Their craft committee is the General Medical Services Committee. Each of these craft committees has responsibilities delegated from the council of the BMA. Each has a regional structure to which local representatives are elected or, in the case of general practitioners, their local medical committee. Non-BMA members are entitled to join in these craft activities.

Local representatives

A parallel BMA structure exists through the largely sleeping regional councils and the more active local BMA divisions. The BMA division nominates place of work accredited representatives (POWARs) who are the professoinal equivalents of shop stewards. They must be BMA members. The POWAR is the first point of contact with the BMA for doctors and can refer problems to its full time regional staff, including the industrial relations officers of the local BMA office. Being a POWAR provides a useful introduction to the BMA organisation with some real prospect of helping your colleagues. The BMA division also elects members to the local joint consultative machinery, which is available only to recognised staff organisations. These local committees do not cover national negotiations, but management should consult them over:

(*a*) strategic planning decisions, including the allocation of resources, which affect staff numbers and jobs;

(*b*) consequent administrative decisions especially those likely to affect the job prospects or job security of particular groups or occupations;

(*c*) all aspects of the immediate work environment, plus those parts of an individual's employment not subject to collective bargaining. This provides interesting insight into union activities and attitudes. In addition the BMA division has representatives on the local health and safety committee.

Each BMA division elects a representative to the annual representative meeting of the BMA. This determines the BMA's broad policies for which the council is the executive body.

There are, therefore, a whole variety of different opportunities for doctors to represent their colleagues' views. Coordination and cross representation ensure some communication between the different parts, but as in any big organisation this is still a real problem. The more active members become, the greater their need to be on several different committees so that their different activities can be linked.

Fellow doctors

The system often needs more doctors as local representatives than there are members who are willing and able to devote unpaid time on behalf of their fellow doctors. Increasingly as the various committees concentrate centrally into smaller numbers, competition for places on them becomes more intense and the proverbial knives come out from time to time. Representation in the medical context means being a representative and not a delegate. There are no card votes. Each representative is elected on his own merits and is entrusted to join in the discussion and debates and to make decisions. The locally expressed view is borne in mind with any new information learnt at the meeting. A delegate has to vote according to the express wishes of the majority of the local group. If the representative clearly departs too far from the views of his or her fellow doctors the democratic process, which often entails yearly elections, allows for his or her prompt replacement.

Doctors' contact with colleagues largely takes place in the course of professional duties, informally over meals, at meetings and postgraduate centres, as well as on the different committees that we all from time to time have to attend, such as the hospital medical staff committee. It is at these encounters that you can gauge the general feelings and attitudes of your colleagues. When contentious issues arise, the discussion level or "grumble index" rises. When you have become a representative on a small national committee or advisory body it is most important to keep in touch with the grass roots, or, as David Bolt, the former chairman of the Central Committee for Hospital Medical Services, put it, with "what the profession would wear." In a brief spell as chairman of the Hospital Junior Staff Committee and during four years as chairman of the negotiating subcommittee of the Central Committee for Hospital Medical Services, I was all too aware of the isolation of such central negotiating bodies.

The strength of the BMA's structure, however, lies in the fact that informed debate at all levels, from medical staff committee, the regional structure, and the different subcommittees of the Central Committee for Hospital Medical Services, tends to run along the same lines. The same arguments and counter arguments are raised and usually the same consensus is reached. This may be a time consuming process but it is helpful in keeping the profession's central representatives in touch with the periphery. I once took a civil servant incognito for a hospital visit which included a canteen lunch at a district general hospital in the south east. Our companions at the table appeared at random, yet the conversation on the current issues was spontaneous and the same as we had been discussing centrally. The day made quite an impression on the civil servant, who admitted that he had never actually visited a hospital. We won our point.

Current issues

A glance at the agenda of the different committees—the local medical staff committee, the Central Review Body Evidence Committee and even the annual representative meetings of the BMA—will show that the same problems recur year after year. On many of the issues there is a balance of opinion and in the cycle of time one or other of the opposite opinions predominates. Any action sets in motion the process of reaction. This has been most notable over the past 20 years with the intractable problem being to resolve the imbalance of medical manpower. Manpower has been an issue that has started many a young doctor on a political career. It seems so simple, just a matter of numbers, until you realise that there are a lot of different factors entailed and that with each the equations become increasingly complex. The main influence is a financial one, which is beyond the profession's control.

The NHS embraced the profession and the profession in turn has become so involved in the NHS that the whole concept of a health service free at the time of use is now part of our medico-political culture. Doctors have become proud and protective of the health service and they invest it with an inordinate amount of good will by working far in excess of their strict contractural duties. Yet doctors are critical, continually asking for more money and better facilities. Their terms and conditions of service specifically allow a practitioner the freedom—without prior consent of the employing authority—to publish books, articles, etc, and to deliver any lecture or speech whether on matters arising out of his hospital service or not. Many modern managers are finding this paragraph difficult to come to terms with. Nevertheless the good will of the medical profession is now a major feature of the service which the changing politicians and the variety of civil servants gaining experience in different departments of the DHSS reluctantly but inevitably come to recognise. Withdrawal of this good will with a work to rule would bring the NHS to its knees. Strike action is unfashionable at present but even in times of great dispute the profession has always shrunk from exercising this right which is now being enshrined as part of a European ethical code. It is always important when such disputes occur to remember that it is the government that has the responsibility for deciding on the level of care provided but it is the doctors who have the duty to care for the patients whom they see irrespective of whether they are in or out of the health service. For the profession, resignation from the service is the ultimate weapon. To strike against patients will lead to the ultimate demise of doctors as professionals.

Ethical issues related to medical practice have become important topics of debate within the profession. Recently, wider political topics have been discussed at the annual representative meeting. In general the public respects doctors' opinions on medical subjects but the further away from medicine itself that the topics are, the less respect that is given to any pronouncements by the BMA. There is a serious danger of alienating patients and devaluing medical opinion if doctors express contentious sentiments about social issues which though relevant are of greater concern to the general body politic.

Skills

The main assets a representative needs are time, patience, and tenacity. Issues always take time to resolve; the latest study leave circular issued by the DHSS appeared after 21 years of negotiations. Occasionally events move fast, which is when experience and wise judgement are needed, and it is important to remember that you never get owt for nowt. Some important skills are needed in committee work and negotiation and recently the BMA has been providing training in these. Such courses provide an important insight into your own abilities, strengths, and weaknesses and if nothing else reduce the number of mistakes you make, thereby ensuring better results in negotiation. These skills can be broadly classified as planning and behaviour. First it is important to find out as much information as possible about a particular topic and decide what the particular issues are. After this you need to canvass opinion and build up a power base by getting support for the objectives from as wide a section of the profession as possible. Then you need to understand the various forces at play in the particular problem you are facing and set ultimate objectives, achievable targets, and the inevitable "fall back" position.

In dealing with other people your professional training comes in useful. You must be able to listen to the various arguments and to hear what others are saying. It is amazing that different participants at meetings can have quite different ideas about what has actually been said. Equally it is very important that any other groups fully understand the nature of what you as a representative are trying to achieve. You must be able to work as a member of a team in any negotiations, with some members doing the talking and others doing the listening. Tension can mount and it is essential to cope with this without losing your cool.

After making representations on behalf of colleagues, it is very important to debrief or undertake a post mortem on the proceedings to see what has or has not been achieved and to keep your colleagues fully informed about the progress of any discussions. Indeed it is the hallmark of a good representative to share ideas and information with those he or she represents so that they in turn can make informed judgements and their views be properly represented.

Is it all worth while?

With the knowledge and support of colleagues our representatives can make progress in improving patient care and defending the independence of our profession, on which the individuality of each patient depends.

The price of freedom is eternal vigilance. It is up to each of us to keep our representatives alert. If you are unhappy about your representative's performance and have the time, toughness, and tenacity, why not try yourself?

Associate with community groups

LILIAS GILLIES

Doctors, like policemen, have traditionally tended to mix only with their own profession. Recently many doctors have come to the view that they must go outside the profession to seek support for their patients' needs. This may be with housing associations to help provide housing for disabled patients, with self help groups who can give support to sufferers of a particular disease, or with groups who might raise funds or otherwise campaign for the development of a service which the doctor and the group agree is needed.

How do you go about it? As secretary of a community health council I suggest that a good starting point is the community health council.

Sounding out

Community health councils recruit at least one third and often more of their membership from voluntary bodies. They also usually make it their business to know and be known by as many voluntary bodies in their area as possible. They have lists of these and their current secretaries which are updated every two years for the election of members of the community health council. So your first port of call could be the community health council office to discuss your project with the staff there who might be able to give you some useful contacts.

The community health council would also be interested in your project because of its interest in improving health services. The easiest first contact is the secretary, and that could lead to some publicity either through a notice given out at the council meeting or inserted in the mailing to council members which usually also goes to a number of local people interested in the Health Service. The mailing from my community health council goes to 150 people who also receive a monthly newsletter, and this is also distributed to health clinics and libraries. A short paragraph in that could identify supporters for your cause.

A council for voluntary service would be able to help with lists of organisations and people to contact, and might also have a newsletter. A volunteer bureau would be able to help with finding volunteers. These organisations are usually aided by grants from the local authority who would be able to supply their addresses. Some hospitals and some social services offices have volunteer organisers who might be helpful. If you work in general practice a patient participation group will be a useful source of people to start self help groups or provide volunteers for helping others.

You might also write a letter to the local newspaper or issue a press release. The free newspapers have the advantage of being delivered to every house.

You may, for example, be a rheumatologist who needs supported housing for people who have become very disabled. There might be a local group such as SHAD (Support and Housing Assistance for People with Disabilities)* interested in such housing to which you could be introduced. They will be glad to have medical advice and a source of clients and you will have a group of people with contacts in housing associations, the expertise for adapting the housing, and the means of providing support.

If you join a committee do attend, if not all the meetings, at least fairly regularly. If you miss a meeting or two keep in touch with the people concerned and the ideas that are being discussed. Contribute to the discussion that you have seen in the minutes with a letter or phone call.

Meeting the public

If there is not an already existing group you will have to set one up. Calling a meeting is the best way to do that. If you have gathered a few interested supporters they will help you. The community health council might help organise the meeting or there might be some other group with related interests such as a dis-

*SHAD, 13/15 Stockwell Road, London SW9.

ability association or league of friends. Community organisations, residents' associations, women's institutes, and townswomen's guilds have regular programmes of meetings and might be willing to have you as a speaker or your project as the topic for one of these.

Having decided to hold a public meeting or been invited to an organisation you must organise what is to happen. If you are not confident that you can hold interest on your own for the whole time is there a suitable film you could use or another more accomplished public speaker? Perhaps it is a new idea or one that has fairly local interest. Then you can add to the interest of your presentation by asking several people to join you on the platform. If, say, you want to start a self help group for patients with cancer and their relatives, you could have a treated patient who is doing well but has to live with the fear of recurrence and a relative of someone who has died. It would be best for the three of you to get together beforehand to talk about what you will say so that it is coordinated. You might find that there is a national group, such as, in this case, Cancer Link, 12 Cressy Road, London NW3 2LY which will be happy to send a speaker along. A national organisation might do all the speaking but it is better if the presentation is made by local people and yourself to bring the subject more directly to the notice of local people.

In preparing for a local public meeting it could help you organise your arguments and get ideas for improving the impact of your project if you go to a conference of a national organisation or a local meeting elsewhere. If you have found some supporters perhaps you could take them with you. You may find that that organisation fits what you want and you could then aim at setting up a local branch. You will in that case benefit from national publicity and national advice. Suppose you want to support the relatives of elderly, confused people. The Alzheimer's Disease Society might fit the bill and you would benefit from the advice of their development workers and could use their publications.* Suppose you want to give more practical help with relief carers. Crossroads Care Attendants might be an organisation that a local group could affiliate to.† You may find that none of the existing organisations meets

*Alzheimer's Disease Society, Bank Buildings, Fulham Broadway, London SW6 1EP.
†The Association of Crossroads Care Attendants Schemes Ltd, 94 Coton Road, Rugby CV21 4LN.

your ideas or the ideas of your group but you can still benefit from them even if you only learn what you do not want.

What do you want?

Having organised your public meeting you should have clear in your mind what you want out of it. If you want to set up a campaign for a new voluntary body you will want a committee. It is best to strike while the iron is hot and collect names of interested people at the meeting. You should invite to the meeting individuals and groups who might have an interest or stand to benefit from your project. If you hope to set up a housing association for people with a mental handicap ask the parents of handicapped teenagers in the local schools and the parents of people in local hospitals for mental handicap who will naturally be concerned about the issue and will have an interest in working towards your aims.

If you want to set up a council on alcoholism (or advisory service on alcohol, which is a more favoured name now) you should also contact social workers, general practitioners, nurses, and probation workers, all of whom are bound to be aware of alcohol misuse among their clients.

Community health councils frequently carry out surveys on a variety of health related topics and might be persuaded to do work related to your project. This could be carried out by council members or students from a local college or Manpower Services community programme or by a paid researcher if money can be raised. This would then provide the focus for a campaign to launch the project. Of course there is always the possibility that the research will show that your favoured project cannot be justified, but that is not likely if you have already done your homework. Nevertheless, research could modify your first thoughts and refine your ideas to meet the community's needs. Though time consuming and not immediately productive, research may be well worth while and should not be neglected. It could go on alongside other developments.

You will need to raise funds for the project. You may in fact only be interested in fund raising for a piece of equipment for your department or an adaptation to a building. Fund raising requires quite a lot of time and preferably a few people to generate ideas and do the letter writing or organising.

One of your earliest objectives should be to get a committee organised so that the amount of time and effort you put in is reduced. Your efforts may produce a group of enthusiasts with time, ideas, and experience to get the project going, raise funds, and cope with the responsibilities of managing the money and staff. What is much more likely is that you will have a few enthusiasts and some of the necessary expertise will be missing. You or the members of the new committee must seek out individuals with the expertise that you require and persuade them to join your committee. The ranks of the newly retired are one of the best groups to recruit from and there are organisations that might help you find the people you need, such as REACH (Retired Executives Action Clearing House)*—which exists to put retired executives in touch with charities that need their particular expertise—or local churches, local Rotary clubs, Lions, or Soroptimists.

Keeping it going

When the committee has done its work and got the project going you must be prepared to take a lesser role. Nevertheless, you must not leave it all to them and thereby have the project move away from your concept and what you perceived as the need. Nor must you direct everything yourself and risk alienating the committee, because they have not got enough to do, and also overworking yourself. Remember that people work best with rewards, so regularly point out the benefits that are coming from the project and endeavour to make sure that everyone feels that they are part of it and are contributing something useful. Social gatherings and celebrations are very important in welding a group together and keeping it going. Training is also important if you are providing a service, particularly one using volunteers.

Associating with voluntary groups may require a lot of unaccustomed effort from you at first but it can be rewarding to you as well as your work, and associating with your patients or their relatives in different ways can be enriching to your practice of medicine as well as to the service to your patients.

*REACH, 89 Southwark Street, London SE1 OHD (01 928 0452).

Run a pressure group and change the law

MADELEINE SIMMS

My own experience of law reform is confined to a quarter of a century's work with a single political pressure group, the Abortion Law Reform Association (ALRA); what I have to say will inevitably be influenced by my experience with this particular cause, which I will draw on for examples to illustrate more general points.

First essentials

Three things are initially required: a clearly defined cause; a group of lively, intelligent, and committed people; and money—preferably lots of it.

A clearly defined cause

The broad aim of ALRA in the early 'sixties when I joined it was clear and straightforward and could be understood without difficulty by everyone: to change the law to enable women to obtain legal and safe abortions more easily. Nevertheless, when a group of lively people get together they are bound to have some differences of opinion, interest, and emphasis. Thus, some of our members simply wanted to extend the medical indications for abortion; others were concerned to introduce social grounds for abortion; others were chiefly anxious to help women avoid giving birth to handicapped babies; while the more radical favoured abortion at the request of the patient. So a degree of consensus needs to be established. People must be prepared to compromise on acceptable minimum aims and to work as a team. Those who demanded too much or were satisfied with two little eventually dropped out or formed their own splinter groups. There is room for all opinions to be expressed, though not necessarily within the same organisation.

A lively, committed, and intelligent group of people

These are the core and lifeblood of any political pressure group. They need to be intelligent in order to recognise the need for reform, to be able to translate it into political terms, and to argue and debate their case in public. They have to be committed because once they are attached to the cause their private lives may cease to exist for a number of years, as flexibility and the ability to seize the moment are of the essence in this kind of political activism. Political crises do not always occur at convenient moments. This means that spouses or partners must also be sufficiently committed to put up with a high degree of domestic disruption. Behind nearly every effective lobbyist there is a long suffering, unflappable, tolerant, and committed partner.

Money and power

In this respect ALRA was largely a failure, as by comparison with the huge sums raised more recently by some religious and antifeminist pressure groups with national networks based on parishes, ALRA had no natural source of either organisation or money other than individual relatively low paid women and the occasional philanthropist—a rare bird indeed. We never solved the problem of money, as successful fundraisers are like gold dust and we were not the sort of fashionable cause likely to attract them. Money is power in politics. It enables you to print elegant, illustrated, easy on the eye literature with a distinctive house style, expounding your cause to many different types of reader. It enables you to take influential political figures out to lunch to put your case in civilised surroundings. It enables you to invite distinguished speakers from far and wide to add their experience to your own on public platforms. It enables you, the committed lobbyist, to travel round the country in reasonable comfort spreading the word, meeting influential supporters, cheering on the troops. It enables you to commission films aimed at a variety of audiences—medical students, women's clubs, schoolchildren, and so on. Lacking the necessary kind of resources and organisation, ALRA members could do only little of any of this, and what they did do was generally undertaken at their own expense—hence the importance of commitment.

The second stage

Having defined the cause, gathered the core of the committee that will run the organisation, and collected such money as is available from well wishers, the next stage is to distribute the jobs.

Who does what

An effective chairman or woman must be elected who commands the total respect of the small group initially assembled, who is clearsighted about the aims, shrewd in assessing the character and available talents of the team, and able to pour oil on troubled waters when this is required—as it often will be in a group of dynamic activists; able also to judge situations coolly and impartially, and to enforce a degree of internal discipline and uniformity when necessary—no small task among a group of unpaid, opinionated volunteers. Such a paragon is hard to find, but because ALRA with singular good fortune did find one in the person of Lady Houghton it was ultimately successful.

Other key posts are that of secretary, who needs to be down to earth, practical, efficient, methodical, and able to use common sense and initiative. The treasurer has the hard and thankless task of trying to raise money from whatever sources might be thought to have some natural sympathy with the cause, and of using whatever is raised to maximum effect. This often puts paid to bright ideas produced by other members of the committee, so the treasurer is not always deeply loved and must not mind this too much. The membership secretary works in close association with both the secretary and the treasurer making sure that membership files are kept up to date and that the particular talents and qualifications of the members are carefully noted in case they are needed, answering queries about membership, ensuring that speakers at meetings remember that recruiting new members is part of their task, and constantly trying to think up new ways of increasing the membership.

There needs to be someone interested in undertaking the research, information, and editorial function, to find out the facts, both historical and current, which have a bearing on the present political campaign and to communicate these to the membership at large so that it can deploy them in local contexts. Thus, some kind of newsletter or house journal is essential for providing information and exchanging news and even gossip.

Two other key officers are required for this committee. One is a press and public relations officer who will mastermind and organise the public aspects of the political campaign, helping to educate the public and being on tap for the media. Publicity stunts and demonstrations may also come into this person's sphere of operations though ALRA in the 'sixties always rather priggishly scorned such activities as being in bad taste and inappropriate to the subject, until members saw with astonishment how effective in crude publicity terms the mass demonstrations of the antiabortion lobby in the 'seventies were.

Finally, the committee needs a political secretary or parliamentary officer who will regularly communicate the views of the association to a group of key parliamentary supporters, feed them with the latest information and statistics which they have not the time to search out for themselves, and write first drafts of speeches for them on request and often at short notice. During parliamentary debates the political secretary has to ensure that enough sympathetic MPs are present in the House to make speeches in support of the cause and are prepared to stay late, even all night if necessary, in order to be present to vote.

Eminent persons and experts

Above and alongside the executive committee are the eminent persons who will serve as presidents and vice presidents and occasionally perform ceremonial, media, or even down to earth advisory functions for the pressure group, and the outside experts who will command respect and influence in the relevant professions. In the 'sixties, ALRA was fortunate in having the loyal and energetic support of one of the most eminent doctors and one of the most distinguished lawyers of their generation in Sir Dugald Baird and Professor Glanville Williams QC, and their active presence encouraged many able young doctors and lawyers to lend their support also. This was long before publicly supporting abortion law reform was considered safe or respectable, when the BMA and the RCOG were still opposed to reform and when *The Times* refused to publish letters in support of abortion law reform even if they merely corrected the inaccurate figures produced by the other side. Only the signatures of VIPs could, on rare occasions, break through this embargo if they were eminent enough or had smart enough addresses such as the House of Lords or the posher gentlemen's clubs. The aspiring social reformer will have to learn the hard way that from the point of view of much of the press it is not what you say that matters, however true or important, but who says it. So having eminent names on tap to append to letters will more than anything else determine whether or not they are printed.

Planning and patience

Once all these officers are installed, they need to draw up a realistic plan of action involving parliament and the media, prepare pamphlets, train speakers, encourage people to write letters to the press, and respond to correspondence from the public. And they need to exercise constant vigilance with regard to the stunts, scandals, and disinformation that opponents will try to perpetrate. In the week before an important parliamentary debate on abortion the gutter press could always be relied upon to produce alarming abortion headlines about "scandals" that generally shrivelled out of sight on closer examination. Meanwhile the damage, in public relations terms, had been done. An educated and informed membership can help to counteract propaganda of this type.

Patience and determination and long term commitment are the essential qualities that social reformers need. In a democratic society changes do not come quickly. Years of public education and public debate precede any major reform. The Abortion Law Reform Association was founded in 1936 by a group of far sighted and courageous women. Only one of them, Alice Jenkins, lived long enough to witness the passing of the 1967 Abortion Act. Fighting for social reform is like planting a great tree. You are unlikely to see the full results in your own life time. It is the next generation that will benefit. So a long view is necessary, as is the conviction that in the very long run rationality and benevolence will prevail.

Further reading

Hindell K, Simms M. *Abortion law reformed*. London: Peter Owen, 1971.

Simms M. Parliament and birth control in the nineteen twenties. *J R Coll Gen Pract* 1978; **28**: 83–8.

Marsh D, Chambers J. *Abortion politics*. London: Junction Books, 1981.

Simms M. The politics of fertility control. *New Humanist* 1981; **96**: 73–5.

Wilson D. *Pressure*. London: Heinemann, 1984.

Set up a patient participation group

TIM PAINE

Patient participation is emerging from its infancy as a new enterprise in general practice. It has become an increasingly common topic for discussion and debate at meetings and conferences, and the number of practices with a patient participation group (PPG) is steadily rising. Although there is still considerable resistance to the idea, especially among long established general practitioners, the number of doctors seriously considering it has multiplied. The principle behind it is as old as the hills: the best results occur when client and craftsman confer over the job to be done and pool their resources in carrying it out. This is the basis of counselling, and patient participation is simply counselling writ large. A PPG is not, and should not be, the only means of participation. Every consultation is an opportunity for sharing—information, insights, solutions and tasks; a PPG is merely a structured and practical method of consultation with the practice as a whole.

What is a PPG? There is enormous variety among the 100 or so in existence, but most share a basic structure. A committee of patients (who may be elected by their peers, or co-opted), together with one of the partners and one or more of the practice team, meet at regular intervals to decide ways and means of making a positive contribution to the services and facilities offered by the practice to its patients. Patient participation group activities tend to fall into five main areas: consumer feedback—a voice in practice planning and organisation; health promotion—meetings, groups literature; community care—various voluntary activities such as transport, fetching prescriptions, and social events; providing information—practice guides, leaflets, local facilities; and fund raising—both to maintain the group and to purchase equipment and provide facilities. By no means all groups engage in all these activities; some prefer to limit their energies to one or two. It very much depends on the interests, priorities, and talents of those concerned and how much time they have to spare. What have practices gained from having a PPG? For many who have become involved—patients and professionals—it is the atmosphere of openness and mutual respect that seems to go with participation that is the most important plus. Others will point to more tangible results, such as a woman partner, a better organised appointments system, or a more congenial waiting room—the results of feedback and suggestions. A health education programme, patient transport service, or lunch club for the elderly are further examples; the list is long. Arguments for having a PPG range from the basically practical (more involvement: better system), to the philosophical (freedom and autonomy) and the political (public service: public say).

Selling the idea

The first task that anybody thinking of starting a PPG should attend to is reading the subject up. This has recently become much easier since the publication of a superb little book by Ann Richardson and Caroline Bray called *Promoting Health Through Participation*.* It is a concise account of the current state of patient participation in the UK, and is a mine of information for anyone about to take the plunge. It is also a valuable guide to publications about patient participation.

If you are inspired by what you have heard and read, and want to proceed, the next step is consultation—with partners, team, and maybe one or two "likely" patients. A large part of this is a selling exercise, and it may tax your powers of persuasion to the full. It is to equip you for this that background reading and thinking are so vital, so that you are sure of your facts and arguments. Of course, the other object of the exercise is to listen to people's reactions and suggestions; "bulldozing" will get you nowhere. One of the reasons groups fail (and this happens not infrequently) is that those concerned have not talked things through sufficiently before they start. This may lead to unrealistic and conflicting expectations, and eventual disillusionment. Do your best to encourage active partici-

* Obtainable from the Policy Studies Institute, 100 Park Village East, London NW1 3SR, price £5.95.

pation from the start. This applies especially to the practice team and staff, who are all too often left out of discussions and plans, and not surprisingly show little interest subsequently. Receptionists and health visitors in particular are valuable allies in the initiation and running of a PPG, and the more opportunity they are given from the start to contribute ideas, suggestions, and their time to the scheme the better will be the prognosis for the group. To make it easier for everyone to gain a clear impression of what a PPG implies, consider inviting one or more people from a thriving group to meet your practice and talk about their experiences. The National Association for Patient Participation (NAPP) comes in useful here. The secretary (Helen Lyus, 13 Manor Drive, Surbiton KT5 8NE) will send you a "start up" package, together with details of contacts in your vicinity.

Once the preliminary discussions are under way, it won't be long before you know if you are on to a winner. It is probably wise to satisfy a few basic criteria before proceeding further: an enthusiastic doctor willing to devote several hours a month, at least initially, to establishing and supporting the group—that's you; partners who are well disposed to the scheme—or at least not antagonistic; one or two members of the practice team who are willing to help enthusiastically; and possibly one or two patients willing to act as catalysts for the first year or two. (You may, of course, decide to delay the involvement of any patients until you are ready for the launch.) Having obtained general agreement, you will need to form a small planning group to examine logistics in detail. Perhaps the most vital aspect to consider is the operational philosophy of the PPG. If you and fellow planners have democracy and accountability at the top of your list of priorities you will probably opt for a committee elected by the practice list and totally autonomous in deciding the range of its activities—so you may decide merely to float the idea at a meeting, describe a few PPG activities and benefits, and let them get on with it. On the other hand, you may want to be a little more directive (in the interests, of course, of PPG effectiveness), and present interested patients with a structure for the group, a list of initial activities and even a constitution. If you veer towards this stance you will need to work out some practical details about how such activities as feedback, health education, and community care might be organised and put into operation.

Funding and publicity can both pose problems. Unless they become very elaborate, PPGs are relatively inexpensive to set up and run. Most groups manage on less than £500 a year, and probably need only £50–100 to get started. Partnerships often contribute this sort of money at the start, and annually thereafter, which is, of course, tax allowable. It is well worth approaching health authorities, particularly if the group is to have a health education role; and local firms and charities are other sources of funds. Once the group is established, it may well become self financing from fund raising activities such as jumble sales, raffles, and sponsored events.

Publicity is probably the biggest headache that you and the group will have to cope with. The constraints on professional advertising are in the process of some degree of relaxation, but it is unlikely that practices will be able to publicise PPG activities other than directly to their own patients. (The one exception is a health education event, which may be widely advertised as long as the practice itself is not identified.) As you will probably be aiming for a maximal response from your patients at the start—most begin with an open meeting to discuss the scheme—it is worth making a supreme effort to circulate as many on the list as possible. This means giving serious consideration to supplementing publicity at the surgery or health centre with a distribution of letters to homes, even through the post. It is also worth putting a lot of thought into how you present your message. The wording and visual impact are crucial, and your planning group may decide that it is helpful to seek some expert advice. Experience has shown that patients respond most positively to communications directly from their doctors, so arrange for the whole partnership to sign the letter before it is duplicated.

When the planning group has done its work, it is wise to have a final practice meeting before the launch, with the proposals and details down on paper. From this stage on it is a good idea to minute discussions and decisions, if only to prevent anyone having an excuse for claiming that they were kept in the dark.

Carrying it through

By this time you and your fellow planners are likely to be somewhat excited and impatient for the huge response to the publicity that you have so carefully engineered. A note of sober caution must be sounded at this point. Patient participation is not everyone's cup of tea, and this applies to patients as well as doctors. So don't be too downcast if only 10 or 20 people turn up to hear more about it. Lots of successful groups have started very modestly. If you have opted for a meeting to promote the scheme (some practices start an activity first, such as a community care scheme, and develop a PPG from there), your presentation and selling skills will again be needed. Try to give everyone who comes a chance to feel involved from the word go. Breaking the meeting up into groups of six or eight, to discuss among themselves what you have just told them (there's no need to move into separate rooms), will get people thinking and enthusiastic. Something that appeals to a lot of people is to feel that they are being given an opportunity to contribute to a worthwhile experiment; there's also a strong tendency to want to make an experiment work. Before the meeting breaks up, you will need to ask for volunteers for the steering committee. Most groups have about 12 patients on their committees, but this may be too many to aim for at the start. Too much arm twisting is usually self defeating in the end, so start small and build up. If you have already found one or two patients who are willing to act as a committee nucleus, it will make things that much easier. The numbers who volunteer will to a large extent determine the range of activities of the group. Avoid being over ambitious; people, including you, will be put off by the number of jobs they have to do. There is, however, an advantage in having a selection of PPG activities. If any prove unsuccessful, the group has other eggs in its basket.

There is often some doubt as to how closely involved the doctor(s) should be in the operation of a PPG once it has commenced activities. My own experience may be relevant. I announced that, having come up with the idea, I now thought it was over to the patients as far as the running of the group was concerned. I felt it was wrong for a doctor to be influencing a scheme set up to give the patients a voice of their own. It wasn't long before the steering committee began to resent my apparent distance from the group, and the lesson I learnt was that you cannot have one sided participation. The compromise, which seems to have worked, was for me, or one of my partners, to attend committee meetings by invitation, and as many of the group's evening meetings as possible. Visible support from doctors goes a long way to maintain PPG morale.

The first year or 18 months of a PPG's life is usually straightforward. Trouble making patients on the committee are seldom a problem; but if they are, their fellow members usually sort them out and they go away without a receptive audience. (I don't mean by this that groups should avoid all criticism of the way the practice is run. Constructive criticism, and coming up with alternative solutions to problems, is part of their raison d'etre.) Once the novelty has worn off to some extent, and the founding members start to feel they have done their bit, a period of doldrums and doubt can overtake a group. New blood is needed, and everyone wonders where it is going to come from. This is a time to inject some extra special effort again, and it may also be worth while at this stage to carry out a pretty honest review of the group's achievements and likely potential; and if everyone agrees it is right to continue, to organise another big publicity drive. Once a group is over this phase of post-honeymoon blues, momentum tends to be maintained. One of NAPP's assets is the opportunity it provides for PPGs in different regions of Britain to meet each other and share experiences. It is a great boost to a struggling group's morale to hear that other people have had similar problems, and have found ways of solving them. One of the commonest frustrations is the unwillingness of patients to participate You have to recognise that it is a minority interest—probably attracting the same proportion of people in a community who might want to attend evening classes. So to achieve a satisfactory response to any meeting, say, one has to make the subject sound relevant to the audience in question, and this again is where skills in communication and "selling" are so valuable.

Setting up a PPG is challenging and exciting, and not without certain risks. One of the refreshing things about PPGs is the lack of standardisation; every practice, and every group, must do its own thing. I have merely suggested a framework, and I am sure no one will feel bound to stick to it. Have a go . . . and good luck.

Be a patient

B T MARSH

I shall be forever grateful to Stephen Potter for his four classic books on how to cope with the vagaries of life, namely, *Lifemanship, Gamesmanship, One-Upmanship*, and *Supermanship*.[1-4] *Lifemanship* was written in 1947, and in my schooldays reading the first three books was de rigueur in the sixth form. In fact you could almost do an "A" level in the subject, and I still find his advice both apposite and welcome some 20 to 30 years later. Many other larger and more erudite treatises on how people react to life have been published over the succeeding years, yet I doubt if any have bettered Potter's acute, albeit exaggerated, observations on how to make the most of one's opportunities and better the opposition, whoever or whatever that may be. I have no intention of making this article a poor man's Potter or an exposition of his various gambits, but I am aware that throughout my experiences of being a patient I have both consciously and subconsciously tried to beat the system with a form of "patientship."

As an opening gambit, "Don't" or "Be lucky" is the best advice I can give to anyone contemplating being a patient, but this fails to take into consideration that most of us have very little choice in the matter. If you are worried about your health it is sensible to consult an expert. Once this consultation begins inevitably you become a patient and are drawn, either willingly or unwillingly, into a whole new world of instability and anxiety, indeed a role reversal with a vengeance. Although I have suggested that you should not be a patient if you can sensibly avoid it, by the same token you should avoid acting as your own physician. This is not because of any doubts about diagnostic competence, as you may get it right, but you may do so for the wrong reasons, in the wrong order, with the wrong conclusion, or with the wrong sense of urgency.

Nobody knows how you feel

I think it important to state that being a patient is an intensely personal experience that we all approach for differing reasons and with differing expectations. Because of this, one thing I have learnt is that no one can truly say, "I know how you feel." Indeed as a patient I became quite angry when well meaning sympathisers made this statement. It is one that should always be associated with some indication that the speaker does not know, but is at least making some attempt to appreciate the situation. This usually prevents the upsurge of anger and frustration that may otherwise be provoked and allows the patient to explain in great detail what he does feel, which certainly helps him, or her, if nobody else.

In June 1984, after a pleasant dinner, I developed severe retrosternal chest pain that was relieved by metoclopramide and antacids. This pain, although less severe, recurred over the next two weeks and was related in my mind to food and to bending. Angina was clearly a differential diagnosis but I was quite unable to provoke the pain by exercise, and it came well below plain indigestion, reflux oesophagitis, and hiatus hernia in my estimation of likelihood. As indigestion was an unusual symptom with me I was eventually persuaded by my wife to make an appointment to see a physician, and I was on the path to becoming a patient. The day before my appointment I had a massive myocardial infarction.

My indigestion had turned out to be oesophageal angina, which has a reputation of being both a mimic and unpredictable. After the infarct I successively underwent cardiac arrest and resuscitation, admission to an intensive care unit, intracardiac pacing, septicaemia, infective endocarditis, insertion of an aortic balloon pump, and, finally, 15 days after the initial event, cardiac transplantation. Discharge home came 12 days later with a convalescence of six months before I returned to work part time, now almost full time. Regular outpatient visits are still necessary (and will be, presumably, for ever) with, at six monthly intervals, an exercise electrocardiogram, a 24 hour electrocardiographic tape, thallium scan, echocardiography, heart muscle biopsy, and, in addition, a coronary angiogram every 12 months. I have described my experiences in greater detail elsewhere,[5] and much of this advice will be specific to these experiences, but I hope that there will be a generic basis that will help those yet to be patients, confirm some of the impressions of those who have been patients, and, for the rest, allow some insight into the feelings of a reluctant but lucky patient.

What is going on

The first thing to realise is that although being in the profession does have many benefits, you are still a pawn to be moved around the chessboard under the aegis of—you hope—a benevolent dictator. Life as a patient is totally different from what you expected, what it was like in your day as a medical student, and what you would like it to be. Day merges into night and nights seem to go on for ever. Time has no relevance and it is quite astonishing how you can lose track of the date and overall time scale. If you are really ill, meals lose their importance at the same time as their taste. This is no reflection on the catering staff, who labour valiantly to excite your appetite. Patients' appetites are still, I think, one of the best indicators of their state of health. Night time sedatives or hypnotics become highly important. Long periods in bed mean frequent naps and consequent difficulty in getting off to sleep at night, with a very light and disturbed sleep pattern, especially in a busy ward or intensive care unit. Judicious use of sedatives helps but a vicious circle is often set up if the sedative is not a short acting one. The patient is then sedated during the morning, often confused, and then becomes even more awake in the evenings.

Even if you have your own room, there never seems to be enough easily accessible space to put things on. Grapes, other fruit, and flowers are, I think, only good for visitors, and "get well" cards are nice to receive but difficult to keep on show. Do not consider your stay in hospital as a chance to catch up on that heavy reading you have been putting off. Solzhenitsyn is definitely out and it will take you all your time to stagger through the most basic newspapers and magazines. A radio cassette player such as a Walkman and, especially, a television with a remote control are absolute musts. The television programmes both entertain—using the word in its broadest sense—and take your mind off your current discomfort. The remote control allows you to jump from station to station as concentration rarely lasts longer than a few minutes, particularly with some of the more erudite programmes.

Information on what is happening to you is often at a premium even though you are in the trade. Do not be frightened to ask what is the real diagnosis and what is the plan of treatment. Invariably you will get a full explanation and be brought into the discussion. It is more difficult, however, to get from your advisers the results of your electrocardiogram, chest radiograph, and other investigations. If you feel aware of what is going on within your body do not hesitate to suggest a diagnosis, particularly if you think that something is going wrong or if you are conscious of a change. You may not be believed and you may be wrong, but at least you should stimulate further examination and thought. Do object if two way conversations occur across the bed between relatives and the attending doctor and you are not included. This is usually inadvertent and arises because it is thought that you are too tired, or sedated, or unwell. Always have your say, as you may want to say "I told you so" at a later date.

Tricks of the trade

There are certain things you should not believe, such as: "It will be just a small prick and it won't hurt"; "We are only going to put in one stitch and there is no need for a local anaesthetic because the injection would be just as painful"; "Everything is fine and don't worry"; "The doctor will be along in a minute"; "You aren't written up for it, so you can't have it"; "We have no idea when you are going to be discharged"; "No, you are not going to be moved from this bed or room"; "You must take this drug, it is essential" (for something that you well know is not essential, such as a vitamin C tablet).

There are other things that you should always ask for if you want them, such as sedatives or hypnotics at night and analgesics if you are in pain or discomfort. Long periods in bed inevitably lead to a tender sacrum and buttocks and an aching back and neck. Despite what some nurses declare, regular massage of the buttocks and sacrum is a tremendous relief, nay, pleasure, even if there is no sign of skin deterioration. A rubber ring and a lambskin undersheet also help to relieve the problem. If you are a male always have at least one spare urine bottle available, and if you have a bedpan ensure that the emergency call button is within easy reach, as sitting on one of these for half an hour is not to be recommended.

A sense of isolation may occur if you are in a room on your own, and the frequent popping in and out of nurses and domestic staff is a great comfort. Needless to say the visit of your spouse plus or minus other sundry relatives and friends is often the highlight of the day. This event becomes so important that at times unreasonable pettiness on the part of the patient can erupt. Comments such as, "Why are you late?" when your spouse has moved heaven and earth to get the family fed and clothed, friends and relatives informed, and other essential jobs performed, are not conducive to harmony. In the same vein, the simple "Thank you" is all that most of the nursing, paramedical, medical, and domestic staff require for the countless small favours that they perform for you during a stay in hospital—it is so easy to say, but so often forgotten.

There are certain essential items that you should take into hospital with you, and tricks that you should know. Always have an adaptor plug set with you. You can bet that the one on the ward doesn't fit, won't work, is lost, or is being used by someone else. Have a mirror with you, preferably a polished metal one. The mirror in the room is rarely in the best spot for shaving, hair drying, or whatever else you are trying to watch yourself do. Have soap, toothpaste, flannel, talcum powder, and other toiletries of your own choice with you, as the make you prefer is never on the trolley. Heels often feel sore after a long period in bed, and it becomes impossible to get your legs in a comfortable position. Ask for a frame to keep the bedclothes off your legs and suggest that someone fills up two rubber gloves with water and ties a knot in the wrist ends. These "donkeys" provide wonderfully gentle supports for the heels, but be prepared for rubber fatigue and a wet bed from time to time. If you have difficulty in pulling yourself up, a knotted rope to the foot end of the bed makes it much easier. Depending upon your particular problem there are many other tricks of the trade that are available—if you ask the right nurse.

Getting out

As you come to discharge time never underestimate the weakness from weight loss and loss of muscle mass that will have occurred if you have been seriously ill and bedbound for some time. You will need help from the physiotherapy department, and this is always readily and efficiently given provided it is asked for or is routine for your type of case. It is remarkable how quickly you can lose strength, particularly for such everyday tasks as getting out of a chair unaided or walking upstairs. This is particularly important, as most bedrooms and bathrooms are on the first floor of a house. This is the time also to ensure that you know exactly what medicine to take, what exercise to perform, and what to avoid when you are discharged. Don't forget to ask what the drill is if an emergency occurs—do you go back to your own general practitioner, ring the consultant, or get yourself admitted to the hospital? When you are being driven home, usually at a sedate 20 to 30 mph, be prepared for this to seem as if you are taking part in a Formula I Grand Prix race. I suggest sitting in the rear seat with your eyes closed.

Finally, a word about outpatients. Find out the critical timings and days associated with your outpatient clinics. Which ones are over booked or under booked, always have plenty of nurses present or appear to be as unpopular with the nurses as they are with the doctors? Is it better to go for radiograph, electrocardiogram, or laboratory tests first or after your consultation? Find out the people who determine the pace of the clinic—what is known in the Royal Navy as "making your number" and in hospital as "getting on the right side of Sister." Ensure that you know the treatment and investigation protocols and then keep a check on these and the results. Familiarity breeds contempt, and minor slips can quickly build up into major problems. When in doubt ask. Follow the instructions unless they appear to be clearly wrong. If they do appear wrong you will often be proved correct. Make a note of your symptoms, reactions, and problems, especially if they are related to something like drugs or food. Pass them on to the physician or nursing staff on your next visit. Much of the lore about a particular condition or its progress is often anecdotal from patients (although many findings get confirmed in the waiting room), and you never know if your experience will be helpful to someone else. If you need regular admissions it is worth while suggesting the most convenient dates for you—surprisingly enough it often works.

Being a patient is a major step that should not be taken lightly. It is an enormous psychological experience that will in most cases entirely change your outlook on life and certainly make you more understanding and sympathetic to other patients. Most patients undergo at least one period of self pity, sometimes many. There is no answer to the querulously put, "Why me?" Each must work out his or her own rationale for what has happened and what will happen in the future. It is also important to realise that your illness might have been equally upsetting to your spouse or relatives and that they may be asking the same questions. Luckily, most people are optimists and although such a question is not unreasonable, it is not too difficult to persuade oneself that all is going to be well. This attitude is essential if there is to be any return to normality. On the other hand, there is no doubt that being a patient can become addictive and may damage your health.

1 Potter S. *Gamesmanship*. London: Hart-Davis, 1947.
2 Potter S. *Lifemanship*. London: Hart-Davis, 1950.
3 Potter S. *One-Upmanship*. London: Hart-Davis, 1952.
4 Potter S. *Supermanship*. London: Hart-Davis, 1958.
5 Marsh B T. A second chance. *Br Med J* 1986; **292**: 675–6.

Work abroad*

ANNE SAVAGE, IAIN WILSON

In times past the decision to work in what was then generally known as "the mission field" required long thought, entailing as it did a lifetime's service, discomfort, isolation, and not a little danger. On the other hand, continuous interesting work was assured. The situation is now reversed, so that easy travel and communications, short contracts, safety, and reasonable comfort must be set against the formidable problems of re-establishment.

When and where

That being so, your first objective if you contemplate spending even a short time abroad must be to secure, as far as possible, your return. Much will depend on your status when you go, but if you are already established on the specialist ladder seek out a sympathetic consultant and discuss your plans; research the possibilities of a future job. The subject of proleptic appointments—that is, those made a year or more in advance—has been more discussed than implemented but a few do exist, and if the demand were articulated more might be created. They certainly bring a sense of security to the troubled mind, but be warned of two possible problems: you may find it difficult, because a replacement is lacking, to return on the appointed date; and you may change your mind. If your ambition is towards general practice then the time spent overseas may count as part of your general professional training but there are no rules, so approach your postgraduate dean. Keep in touch while you are away, and keep a log of interesting cases. It will provide

---

* This is an expanded version of the chapter with the same title by Anne Savage in *How To Do It* Vol. 1, 2nd ed.

fascinating reading for your old age, and may prove useful before that as evidence of experience and ability. Do not neglect research. The Third World is so full of unexplained problems that a reasonable project could be devised and carried through, even in the absence of sophisticated equipment.

When to go is mostly a matter of circumstance, but those in a position to choose might consider the following points. It is easier to study and pass examinations if you continue in an unbroken succession of posts; you will get more out of your time spent abroad if you are already some way up the professional ladder. This applies especially to surgeons and obstetricians; you may be able to incorporate your overseas appointment into your training programme. As mentioned before, this mostly applies to general practitioners, but a few specialist accredited posts exist. Inquire at the appropriate royal college if in doubt; if, as is possible, experience of other disciplines leads to a wavering in your dedication, a move is more easily made at an early stage; if you have children their education must be considered. Up to the age of 7 the local school will serve; after that the cultural differences become sharper, and apart from a few good international schools the choice lies between boarding school and home tuition.

Where to go? No problem as to country because of the global shortage of doctors. Avoid South America unless you are proficient in Spanish or Portuguese. Parts of Africa are francophone, otherwise the lingua franca is English. Religion rarely causes problems, statements such as "strong Christian commitment" being self explanatory, but many mission and ex-mission hospitals, even when staffed by religious orders, accept recruits of all faiths or none. Race may occasionally deter: Asians are not accepted in some African countries and some African nationals may not travel to South Africa. Consider carefully the type of hospital, often designated by the number of doctors on the establishment (not necessarily the number in post at any one time), and unless you are very self confident and a handy general surgeon avoid the one doctor ones. Promises of back up by a nearby centre are worthless if the only road has been washed away by rain.

Paperwork

A choice made, set about getting your papers. In almost all cases a work permit and registration with the medical council are necessary; most often you will need your papers on entry to the country, but occasionally they may be handed over at the airport, or even some time after your arrival. Forms can be voluminous and forbidding. They are devised by the public service departments with the object of sifting out the dross, of which a fair bit floats round the Third World. Do the best you can: details of your kindergarten successes are not necessary if you have completed university education, but do read the small print, and remember that a commissioner for oaths is not necessarily a notary public, and only the latter may certify some photocopies.

At the same time write direct to the medical superintendent or a senior doctor. Sending agencies cannot be expected to be fully up to date, and departments of health are often very vague—and sometimes positively misleading—about conditions at the periphery. It is as well, before the wife and children step wearily into their new home, to make sure it has some furniture and means of cooking. In addition to the basic questions—housing, shops, schools, and recreational facilities—make a list of the smaller things that might cause problems: voltage, refrigeration, radio reception, availability of any regular medicines, and contraceptives. Do not forget a car. Public transport is mostly overcrowded and unreliable, and taxis are scarce, expensive, and rarely used by the cognoscenti. A second hand vehicle may be available. If not, with an eye to spares, find out which make is more favoured locally, or arrange for a supply from home. Consult the tax office or an accountant and perhaps the relevant chapter in that excellent publication *Brits Abroad*[1] for guidance in the maze of regulations governing the position of expatriates. You may wish to let your home; consider well the effect that that might have on your tax and mortgage position. Make a will; give somebody in the United Kingdom access to sufficient of your assets to pay subscriptions and unexpected bills. Inquire of the royal colleges, General Medical Council, and defence societies about possible reductions in subscriptions.

If a lengthy, unnerving silence follows your application write again. Funding, a familiar problem, is even more so in developing countries, and if the budget is overspent all posts may suddenly be frozen. When your documents come check carefully not only details of salary, conditions, and length of employment, but also possible allowances—settling in, clothing, etc—or tax free advances of salary. Finally, do not forget insurance, both personal and for your

British possessions, and arrange it in the UK if possible. In the event of a claim there are advantages in settling in sterling.

Look forward

Between decision and departure gather as much information as you can. Medical superintendents desperate for staff may paint a rosy picture and make extravagant promises. Forewarned is fore-armed, not necessarily frightened off. Contact with somebody recently returned is invaluable, and students on electives, in particular, can be the source of unbiased and uninhibited comment. Start making lists. Little things mean a lot when you are miles from the nearest shop and even further from "civilisation." Old *BMJs* may serve as toilet paper; nothing substitutes for soap.

It is easier to settle if you know something about the country, its history, and people. Hunt the libraries and consider attending a course. Some professional preparation is advisable, though it is comforting to realise that even in the tropics most of the patients will be suffering from "European" conditions. Books and audio-visual aids are helpful for those unable to attend a formal course, and informal education may be arranged in the host country. Fortify yourself against cultural deprivation by taking or arranging for the supply of cassettes and any hobby materials. Most import-antly, if travelling as a pair, one of whom is not medically qualified, consider the role of the partner. It is essential that he or she be actively involved and a willing participant. Failure to resolve this problem has led to contracts, sometimes the marital one, being prematurely terminated. As with so many aspects of Third World living the difficulty is more psychological than real, for in places where talent is so short anyone healthy, flexible, and willing will be pressed into service.

Flexibility is indeed the most important quality to take with you. Couple it with a degree of circumspection, particularly with regard to politics. Although it is true that the major problems of the world will only be solved by political action, this is not true at the local level where partisanship may divide, alienate, and ultimately de-stroy all you have attempted. You may find the local people watch-ful and uncommunicative at first, so learn enough of the language and customs for basic courtesy. Failure to greet formally or shake hands may be greatly, if silently, resented. The reward for this slight trouble will be genuine friendship. In the hospital honesty is the only policy. If you don't know something, say so. Medical cowboys, like medical tourists, are distrusted and resented, and, except in a few establishements still boasting long serving medical superintendents, information is rarely "de haut en bas," more an exchange between peers.

Most of the anxieties that afflict intending travellers disappear on arrival. Perhaps a few can be dispelled here. With the exception of areas of war or anarchy you will probably be safer than in the UK, and there, as here, the main danger is from traffic accidents. Given adequate prophylaxis against the obvious hazards—malaria and so on—the incidence of disease is probably much the same, gastroenteritis replacing respiratory incidents in the rich tapestry of daily life. Do not fear being stranded: help and hospitality are universally to be found. New techniques are easier to learn when the mystique that surrounds so much British apprenticeship is dispelled. If, after sufficient time for mutual adjustment, incompatabilities persist, transfer to another hospital can usually be arranged.

Finally, in times of doubt and uncertainty, cling to two undoubted facts: far more doctors working overseas stay on after the end of their contract than return prematurely; and many who originally came as students or immediately after registration later return as mature doctors. In fact your main problem may be, in more than one sense, adapting back.

Prepare for a sabbatical year in the United States

R W TALBOT

Negotiating the early morning traffic wending slowly into London, I thought it a good time to consider my future: second year senior registrar in surgery, MS, two to six years to a consultant appointment. Why not take sabbatical leave and fulfil my ambition of spending a year in the United States?

In this chapter I have attempted to summarise the organisation required before I set off for Gatwick Airport 10 months later, in the hope that it might be of value to other potential travellers.

Appointment

The decision where to go will be guided by your clinical and research interests and the availability of personal contacts. It is important to allow a month for replies to postal communication and to use the telephone as much as possible. The director of the host department will play an essential role in obtaining institutional approval, initial planning of any projects, and possibly funding, but it is essential to contact the administrator designated to foreign medical graduate programmes. With a direct telephone number for this person most problems can be solved rapidly and without weeks of delay and worry.

Initial travel matters

Visa

Visa qualifying examinations are administered by the Educational Commission for Foreign Medical Graduates (3624 Market

Street, Philadelphia, Pennsylvania 19104–2685; tel 215 386 5900). The educational commission's medical test no longer meets visa requirements and has been discontinued. The visa qualifying examination retains its equivalence with the current Foreign Medical Graduate Examination in the Medical Sciences provided the educational commission's English test has been passed within the previous two years.

The Foreign Medical Graduate Examination in the Medical Sciences is a two day examination in basic sciences and clinical sciences. The basic science test can be taken any time after completion of the basic science curriculum at a medical school listed in the *World Directory of Medical Schools*. The clinical science test can be taken within one year of completion of the full clinical curriculum. These two tests can be taken separately or together.

The Foreign Medical Graduate Examination in the Medical Sciences is required for a visa to undertake a "hands on" or clinical appointment, but no exams are necessary for research or observation appointments. Once the appointment and funding have been secured the institution in which the appointment will be held or the sponsoring institution in the United States will initiate the application for a J–1 exchange visitor visa. When the documentation has been processed the certificate of eligibility (IAP–66) will be forwarded to the "alien physician"

Once you have received this certificate and evidence of funding and of re-employment on return to the United Kingdom, have completed an application form for a temporary non-immigrant visa (form 156, available from most travel agents or the United States Embassy) for each member of the party, and have a passport size photograph for all applicants aged 16 and above and a British passport valid for at least six months after the date of return, you can obtain the visa by post or in person from the local visa branch of the US Embassy (England and Wales: Visa Branch, US Embassy, 5 Upper Grosvenor Street, London W1A 2JB. Scotland: US Consulate General, 3 Regent Terrace, Edinburgh EH7 5BW. Northern Ireland: US Consulate General, Queens House, 14 Queen Street, Belfast BT1 6EQ).

Other members of the party will receive a J–2 dependant's visa and will not be allowed to work unless they can change their visa once in the United States on grounds of financial hardship. Ideally, if other members of the family want to work while in the United States they should obtain an appointment and visa in advance.

163

Travel grants

It is not difficult to secure an appointment, but funding by the institution will not always be available. Research grants may be available through your own institution or from other sources mostly managed by or through the Medical Research Council. Advice on funding should initially be sought from your own department.

Facilities are available to help with travelling expenses, and many of the royal colleges have their own bursaries or funds endowed by medical industries. Other funds exist and are advertised in the *BMJ* and *Lancet* and include the King Edward's Hospital Fund for London. Many of these bursaries and research grants must be applied for 18 months or more in advance. I found the direct approach to pharmaceutical companies particularly unrewarding.

It is a good idea to save four to six weeks of annual leave for embarkation. This provides an overlap in salary to cover the initial period in the United States. It is an additional comfort having your final salary paid into your depleted United Kingdom bank account after departure.

Financial matters

Tax

A tax consultant is essential because the tax status of British subjects abroad is complex and not easily gleaned from the Inland Revenue. When a person works abroad for one or two years his salary is not subject to United Kingdom income tax provided visits home do not exceed the maximum allowed. Caution is advisable when working abroad for only one year to be certain that a full year has been completed. Taking annual leave at the end of an appointment to return home can make the salary liable to tax.

Article 20 of the tax treaty between the United Kingdom and the United States may be of benefit. It states that, "if a teacher or researcher who is a resident of one country is invited to teach or engage in research in the other country, he will be exempt from tax by the host country on income from teaching or engaging in research if he is present in that country for a period not expected to exceed two years. If the two year period is exceeded, the exemption will be lost retroactively." Some research grants specifically exclude this exemption, and many employing authorities are unaware of it.

Tax deductions on mortgage interest paid at source (MIRAS) can continue while you are abroad, although the Inland Revenue initially denied this. It was valuable to transfer all these problems to a tax consultant, whose fees were partially tax deductible.

Health insurance

Health insurance is prohibitively expensive to arrange in the United Kingdom, costing a minimum of $300 per person for one year, and it should be unnecessary. Medical institutions in the United States run staff health schemes that include all members of the family, and it is wise to confirm this in advance. These schemes provide full health coverage at very reasonable rates (we paid £40 a month for the whole family).

It is advisable to take out travellers' insurance to cover the first few days before taking up your appointment.

Home finance

National insurance—depending on when in the fiscal year you leave the United Kingdom and for how long it may be unnecessary to pay contributions. The Department of Health and Social Security booklet *Social Security Abroad* (N138), available from any local office of the DHSS, gives full details, which should be confirmed by writing to the DHSS Overseas Branch, Newcastle upon Tyne NE98 1YX.

Superannuation—When taking sabbatical leave it is important to ensure that the employer's superannuation contributions are continued by the employing authority in the United Kingdom. On return home the employee's contributions can be paid retrospectively over six months.

Family allowance—The DHSS booklet *Child Benefit for People Leaving Britain* (CH6), available from any local DHSS office, outlines the position for families abroad. Family allowance may still be received during an absence of one year or less, but this information is far from clear and it is worth sending an application to the DHSS Overseas Branch even if eligibility seems unlikely.

Medical indemnity organisations will not insure doctors against malpractice while they work in the United States, and if notified they will suspend membership and hold the premium in credit. Indemnity for the period before departure continues unaffected. Most academic institutions in the United States will provide this insurance for those engaged in clinical work. Some colleges and organisations have reduced subscriptions for members abroad, and many journals have distribution agents within the United States.

Banking—It is important to discuss plans with the bank, who can advise on payment of bills and transfer of money to and from the USA and make provisional plans for overdraft facilities if these are likely to be required. Money can be taken to the United States either as a bank draft in dollars or as travellers' cheques. Credit card companies will send accounts direct to the bank for payment if requested to do so or to the United States for payment against a United Kingdom bank account or in dollars. Credit cards are difficult to obtain without a "credit rating" on arrival in the United States, but the local bank can usually overcome this. There is an annual charge of up to £25 for each credit card.

Savings accounts—In most cases long term saving accounts with banks and building societies pay higher interest than accounts giving easy access. Transfer of money not required into one of these accounts or preferably into savings not taxed at source will be advantageous.

Property

Letting property is complex and fraught with pitfalls. It is essential to consult a solicitor and preferably to employ an agent, despite fees of 15–20%, to manage the tenancy. If the property is mortgaged the building society or bank must be informed in advance of plans to let, and it may insist that an agent be employed. It will also want to view the tenant's references.

Service contracts should be arranged for large appliances—for example, boilers and washing machines. The owner is responsible for rates and water rates, which can be paid by direct debit. Household insurance companies reduce their liabilities when the property is let and exclude breakages, damage, and theft by tenants. The terms of existing policies should be clarified. A good agent will arrange transfer of services and telephone into the tenant's name and will arrange payment of final accounts. Post should be redirected by the Post Office, preferably to someone who will handle routine correspondence and forward important letters. The agent will provide lists of furnishings required in the house, and some time should be spent preparing the house and garden. It is worth remembering that the tenant will expect everything to be in perfect working order, and repairs that the tenant initiates will invariably be more expensive than if they had been carried out before departure.

It is inadvisable to leave items of monetary or sentimental value for use in the house. Small items can be secured in a cupboard or stored with relatives, but do not forget to confirm that they are still insured. It is difficult to decide what to take to the United States, but the voltage and cycle (120 V,60 C) are different and most electrical appliances are incompatible without expensive stepdown transformers for high wattage appliances. Most small appliances can be purchased cheaply and sold at "garage sales" before you return home.

Travel arrangements

Obtaining a visa has already been covered. It is advisable to have children included on both parents' passports in case separate travel home may be required.

Apex and charter flights are not available for periods exceeding six months, but discounts of up to 15% can be obtained on regular single or open return flights by shopping around, particularly by checking advertisements in travel magazines. There is a temptation to fly with cheaper carriers to New York—for example, People's Express or Virgin Atlantic Airways—and to fly on from there, but the ultimate small savings over direct flights are often far outweighed by the time taken and inconvenience. It is important to realise, especially when travelling with children, that baggage must be retrieved and cleared through immigration and customs at the first airport of landing, even if onward flights are with the same carrier.

There are advantages in buying an open return ticket, especially if you have a grant towards travel costs. Single air fares from the United States are generally higher than those bought in the United Kingdom. The open return, however, is valid for only 365 days, which is too short to allow you to work a full year and avoid tax liability on the return home. We took the risk of buying return tickets and persuaded the carrier to extend them for a few weeks at no extra cost. Nothing is lost by trying because return tickets can be traded in for their full cost price.

Excess baggage charges are lower than air freight, so if the standard baggage allowance is inadequate check these charges, and restrictions on weight and dimensions, with the carrier.

Driving and accommodation

An international driving licence is not essential but is advisable because it contains a stamped photograph. Driving licences are used as identity cards in the United States, especially for cashing cheques. For a stay of longer than one year a local driving test would be required. Membership of the Automobile Association allows you to receive reciprocal services from the American Automobile Association and is a little cheaper. As a member of the American Automobile Association, however, you can obtain a Visa card without the annual £15 charge and free travellers' cheques, which are useful for travel within the United States

Furnished apartments may be available, but rented houses in the United States are usually unfurnished, although they may contain kitchen appliances (that is, oven, fridge, and washing machine). Furniture can be rented separately, but it is fairly easy to furnish a house from the many garage sales and through small advertisements in local newspapers. Most large institutions have their own sales and rent newspaper through which accommodation might be arranged in advance.

The immediate neighbourhood of large city hospitals is not always safe or desirable. It is not essential to arrange accommodation in advance, but if you are determined to do so a preliminary visit, finances permitting, or, at the very least, advice from a local resident, is essential. If a liaison can be established with people returning to the United Kingdom exchange of accommodation, car, and furniture en bloc might be beneficial. In larger cities the quality of public schools (state schools) may vary widely and be an important factor in determining where to live.

For families with children I strongly advise against rushing into a furnished apartment. A little time and effort spent furnishing a house will pay dividends both in home comfort and in enabling you to meet other families, which is vital for domestic harmony.

Second hand cars can be bought cheaply but may turn out to be expensive to run. A newer and more expensive car can be acquired by leasing, which has the added advantage of leaving you capital with which to furnish the house.

In short, the message is to take as much money as possible and arrange for a loan or advance in salary if necessary. In the first three weeks we spent £3800 setting up home, which included a £1000 returnable deposit on the house and car lease.

Children

Before leaving ensure that your children's school holds a place for them on return. A résumé of the reading level and general academic grade of the children is helpful in placing them in school, especially if they are under 6. American children start school at 6–6½, but schools will usually accept foreign children who have started school at home.

Inoculation against measles, mumps, and German measles in addition to diphtheria, pertussis and tetanus, and polio may be required before admission to school, but this can be arranged on arrival.

Lectures

Prepare a couple of seminars, with slides, on any original work or investigation previously performed. In addition, slides of British cities and countryside are worth having for informal lectures, to show at the children's school and to friends.

Departure

Transatlantic flying is no longer romantic, especially when you are travelling with children. Try to reserve seat numbers in advance and telephone again on the morning of departure to reinforce the request and thereby avoid the all too frequent attempts to separate families on aircraft. Motel accommodation for the first night and transport from the airport can be arranged in advance with local advice.

With advance planning a period abroad can be painless and enjoyable.

Take a sabbatical from general practice

IAN TAIT

The secret of success in achieving a sabbatical from general practice is sufficient motivation. If you want to do something enough you will surely find a way to do it—or die in the attempt. Taking a sabbatical shouldn't end like that but there will always be difficulties to overcome, and a momentum has to be maintained if the bags are really going to be packed, the farewells said, the dog found a home, and the front door closed for real.

Motivation can be entirely self generated but it helps a lot if others share your commitment. The people you really have to win over are first and foremost yourself, then your family, and then your practice. Once that is done there will be other practical difficulties concerning authorities and agencies, but none of these is likely to defeat you, though they may annoy and delay you.

Convincing yourself

Why take a sabbatical? I think there are overwhelming reasons why doctors working in general practice should have a sabbatical period working or studying away from their practices. General practice is for most of us a long service affair. In the early years we have a lot to stimulate and challenge us: we have to settle into our practice and build it as near to our heart's desire as we can, and come to terms with the result. After that there is often little outward change to provoke a fresh surge of interest and energy. The "burn out" syndrome is beginning to be recognised as a real problem in the middle and late years of a general practitioner's professional life. When this happens most of us soldier on, but it can be a disenchanted business and leads all too easily to apathetic time serving, which is bad for the doctor, his practice, and his patients. Some take to alcohol or love affairs, but a safer remedy is to take sabbatical leave. I believe that this should be thought of not as an optional extra but as a necessary part of our professional lives—just as it is in universities and academic departments; and of course the reason is the same. Academics, once they have tenure, are locked in a system which is unlikely to change for many years. They too are in danger of growing stale and unproductive, and it is for this reason that they are offered—and often required—to take sabbatical leave. General practitioners should do the same.

The doctor's family

A doctor's family will need to prepare itself in all sorts of ways if it is to make the best use of a period of sabbatical leave. More plans for taking a sabbatical come to grief because of the disruption it threatens to cause to the lives of other members of the family than for any other reason. There needs to be a lot of honest communication and a willingness to compromise. But with enough warning and enough thought the sabbatical can and should be a rewarding experience for all.

Convincing the practice

If we really believe, as I think we should, that a sabbatical period is an important part of our professional life, then it should be discussed and agreed in principle with the practice. This should happen long before there are specific plans for any particular individual to take sabbatical leave. Some practices write sabbatical arrangements into their partnership contracts. It would be good if this became the rule rather than the exception. Matters that need to be covered in such agreements should include: when partners are entitled to take sabbatical leave, and for how long; how the work is to be covered, particularly the employment of locums; and what financial arrangements are acceptable. One large practice I know always has one of its partners on sabbatical leave. We should take advantage of the surprising degree of freedom given to us under our terms of service.

Financial aspects

The question of the expenses entailed in locum cover for a

sabbatical leave is likely to be the single most important factor in deciding what you do with your sabbatical. If you are to be personally responsible for the cost of providing a locum, you will probably need to take paid work. This can turn out to be something of a busman's holiday. Traditionally the idea of a sabbatical does include a sense of unpressurised time and freedom from the need to earn one's keep by daily toil—a chance to stand back and take stock. We should try to preserve this ideal; it is not impossible, as has been proved by those practices that have achieved arrangements to cover partners on sabbatical leave, thereby giving the departing doctor freedom to do something that really interests him.

Theory into practice

Given that the ground work has been done and you have reached the stage of deciding what to do during your sabbatical, what are the options open to you?

Extended study leave

Arrangements for granting extended study leave to general practitioners exist under the terms of our contract with the DHSS. The guidelines and administrative conditions that apply to study leave are described in SFA 50.1 to 50.4. Applications need to be approved by the postgraduate dean of the region in which the doctor works, via the GP regional adviser and the GP subcommittees of the regional postgraduate committee. It is best to consult your GP regional adviser, who will give advice on how to apply and surmount the various bureaucratic hurdles. Final approval is needed by the DHSS. To quote its own words:

In all cases the over-riding considerations will be whether a doctor's application for prolonged study leave is in the interests of medicine in a broad sense, or otherwise in the interests of the Health Service as a whole.

This definition is annoyingly vague. It means, in theory at least, that the scope of "work" is very wide, though in practice it seems that applicants may have to argue their case with some skill. It is difficult to establish any guidelines for acceptability. If successful the doctor will receive an educational allowance (currently about

£34 a week). The regulations also allow for the payment of locum expenses; these used to be paid for any doctor, but the DHSS now applies rules similar to those applied to locum payments for doctors who are absent during sickness. Thus doctors with relatively small lists may find that they are in fact not entitled to locum expenses—so check this side of things before you disappoint yourself and your practice. Study leave can be taken for any period between 10 weeks and 12 months.

Exchange of practices

Some doctors have, through personal contacts, exchanged practices with doctors in other countries. Obviously these arrangements remove problems with locum cover. So long as the personalities concerned are compatible this can be a very good way of gaining a different perspective on medical practice. The difficulty seems to be that integrating the different needs of two doctors and their families can be very complicated. It also has to be said that regulations governing the right to medical practice in different countries, and even different parts of the same country, seem to get more complex and more restrictive. Anyone considering an exchange with another doctor would need to be very careful to check this side of things.

Locum or short term work

The range of locum work that may be available to a British doctor seeking sabbatical experience is less extensive than it was, but employment is still available as follows:

GP locums—There are agencies that arrange for the employment of British doctors in some countries—for instance, Canada, Australia, and New Zealand. Such agencies will undertake to employ doctors for a definite period. There may be some registration problems in parts of Canada but this does not yet seem to be a problem for work "down under." Being a locum is not likely to be a relaxed holiday. My partner is currently doing a locum sabbatical near Brisbane, and his last letter reported seeing 60 patients a day. One cannot help feeling that the easier locum jobs get filled locally, and agencies advertising abroad are often trying to fill unpopular slots.

Work with international companies—Medical posts with companies working abroad or for medical services in the Middle East are advertised regularly in the *BMJ*. Conditions of service should, however, be scrutinised carefully.

Medical recruitment by the government's Overseas Development Administration is now much reduced. My partner and I gained contracts to work in Swaziland for 18 months each, but that was more than 20 years ago. Work is still available, however, and a local colleague spent three months of 1985 working in the Falklands, where he had lived as a young boy. Such contracts are usually only given for longer periods, but special situations allow for negotiations, and it is always worth a try.

Voluntary, semivoluntary, and mission work—Where medical needs are great, work can still be found. This generally means that no local medical resources can be found to do the job. Organisations seeking the help of British doctors in this way include mission hospitals, relief agencies such as the Red Cross, Oxfam, and Save the Children Fund, and voluntary agencies such as Voluntary Service Overseas. Those seeking this kind of work should contact reliable organisations for information—for instance, Christians Abroad, International Voluntary Service, or the Bureau for Overseas Medical Service. Addresses and telephone numbers are given at the end of the chapter.

In general it will be easier for doctors to find work if they possess some extra skills, such as basic surgery, anaesthesia, or operative obstetrics. Also in demand are proved skills in health care education. For those considering this kind of work the Bureau for Overseas Medical Service organises occasional short courses to teach basic surgical and other special skills. On another level there is a need for doctors willing and adaptable enough to survive in primitive conditions in isolated areas. This would hardly apply to a middle aged British doctor with a family.

The question of length of contract is often a difficulty. Most organisations prefer contracts of one or two years, but shorter contracts are available. Action 2000, organised from Addenbrooke's Hospital, Cambridge, specifically sets out to cater for doctors offering shorter terms of service—for example, three to six months—as well as longer contracts.

Doing your own thing

Refreshment of spirit seems to me to be the major justification for taking a sabbatical and depriving our patients of our services. We may find ourselves doing the same kind of work as we usually do, though in another setting, but perhaps we should try to do something different—to adopt for a while a new rhythm of life, and perhaps a different identity. I spent a truly recreative year working with the Wellcome Unit of Medical History at Cambridge; others whom I know have become serious research workers for the first time, journalists, travellers, or explorers. Others have taken to the arts, music, painting, writing, potting, or other crafts.

Travel grants, scholarships, awards, etc

Although these are unlikely to cover the expenses entailed in taking sabbatical leave, they can help. They can also serve as a useful passport for a doctor when visiting other doctors or institutions by lending some sense of academic credibility to the visitor.

The bodies offering awards include the British Medical Association, Royal College of General Practitioners, and the World Health Organisation. Research grants are available from regional health authorities, the DHSS, and from independent bodies such as the King's Fund, or the Nuffield Foundation. Finally, an increasing number of drug companies offer awards that could form the focus for a period of study on sabbatical leave—for instance, the Schering Scholarships for GP trainers, currently worth £1000.

Re-entry and splash down

I do not think I should end these thoughts on taking a sabbatical leave without some reflection on the return to work in the practice. To the extent to which the sabbatical has been successful you will have changed. You will not be quite the same doctor, or even perhaps quite the same person, who left the practice. No one should expect to find the re-entry easy. This process is not helped by partners and patients who expect you to be all instant eagerness and fresh energy. As a returning traveller, will find that everyone else in the practice has fixed their holidays in the confident expectation that you won't really need one. You should not despair. Your sabbatical will, I hope, have stored up treasures for you which will become their own reward once the readjustment is over.

Occasionally, of course, the sabbatical is the occasion for a necessary self examination that provokes a major change in the direction of your professional life. If so, so be it. It is good that such changes should be made while time is still on our side. Otherwise we are in danger of joining what Thoreau thought to be the majority of men, who "lead lives of quiet desperation." So if you haven't already done so, start planning your sabbatical now—and don't forget to tell your partners and your spouse.

Useful contacts for sabbatical employment

Bureau for Overseas Medical Service (BOMS)
Africa Centre
38 King Street
London WC2E 8JJ
Telephone: 01 836 5833
Administrator: Jane Lethbridge

Christians Abroad
11 Carteret Street
London SW1H 9DL
Information secretary: Deborah Padfield

Action Health 2000
35 Bird Farm Road
Fulbourne
Cambridge CB1 5DP
Telephone: 0223 245252 ext 7466 (2–5 pm)
Director: Dr M Kapila

Overseas Development Administration
Crown Agents
4 Millbank
London SW1P 3JD
Inquiries to the recruitment executive

Voluntary Service Overseas (VSO)
9 Belgrave Square
London SW1X 8PW

International Voluntary Service (IVS)
53 Regent Road
Leicester LE1 6YL

Oxfam
274 Banbury Road
Oxford OX2 7DZ
Inquiries to the disaster emergency officer

Save the Children Fund
Mary Datchelor House
17 Grove Lane
Camberwell
London SE5 8RD

British Red Cross Society
9 Grosvenor Crescent
London SW1 7ET

Retire: 1

DAVID WALDRON SMITHERS

There are no rules. Thankfully no two people are the same, so it is impossible to impart any formula for retirement; it is an enterprise that each must plan and carry out for himself. Nevertheless, some thoughts on a change which may turn out to be a predicament or a jubilation, a deprivation or an indulgence, a shock or a planned enhancement of living, may set the mind to work on the subject, if only in tabulating omissions or in angry disagreement.

Get ready for it

One thing is certain, namely, that the best advice about retirement is "Be prepared." Leon Trotsky in his *Diary in Exile* wrote that "Old age is the most unexpected thing that ever happens to a man." It certainly does tend to creep up on the retired. There are plenty of books about such preparation and a magazine called *Choice* which offers help to those about to come to grips with it. Taking first things first: being financially padded as far as the available resources will allow for the foreseeable future will not cause any problem to vanish but will make nearly all of them seem less pressing. For those who do not command financial wizardry, the British Medical Association runs investment, tax, and retirement planning seminars for members and spouses—who are offered lunch as well for £10 each—that set about these fundamentals at remarkably low cost.

Perhaps "When" should not intrude on a "How" article, but there are a few doctors—among such branches of medicine, for example, as ophthalmology, dermatology, or general practice—who are able, if they wish, to continue in practice into their 80s and so never really retire at all. This I understand, though it seems a sad waste of a wonderful opportunity. So "Why" enters the lists at times. I once sat next to a courtly, balding, white haired surgeon at an introductory tea ceremony in a Canton hospital, who presented his colleagues to us in Chinese through an interpreter and then turned to me, speaking faultless English, to say that we did not understand retirement in Britain. He said that he no longer operated but, for as long as he wished, he would take some outpatient sessions and do some teaching. He then added, with sparkling glee, "and I am on full salary."

For most of us "When" is 65—still time to start a new career, if a little late. Sir Harold Himsworth has become a philosopher, but I suppose he always was one. In my time I have advocated a series of most sensible changes in medical and nursing practice, generally regarded as totally impracticable. My notion on retirement was that the heads of hospital departments should abandon their administrative responsibilities in their 50s to allow younger people to plan the future they will have to cope with. Older consultants, happily freed from a great deal of planning and committee work, would then be better able to deploy their hard won experience, so valuable both in practice and in teaching. Whenever the time does come for retirement, however, it would be wise to listen to Alexander Pope:

> You've play'd and lov'd and eat and drank your fill.
> Walk sober off before a sprightlier age
> Come titt'ring on, and shove you from the stage.

Natural breaks

In retirement there are some dangers to avoid. One of these is to go on too long speaking at meetings; medicine advances fast today, doctors can soon get out of date on retirement, and most junior colleagues are kindly people who will applaud and keep you in the dark because you were once worth listening to. Another danger is to cut yourself off too suddenly from caring for others; personal or community care is in a doctor's bones and an unhappy feeling of being useless after a lifetime of service can be quite distressing. Another danger is embodied in a proposal to move from home. If this is the plan you would be wise to spend as much time as possible at the new location well in advance of the move. A sudden separation from friends and familiar surroundings, even to a lovely place in the sun or, as, in Plato's retirement, "Where the Attic bird trills her thick-warbled notes the summer long," does not always work out too well and seldom comes up to expectation without careful preparation. It was a doctor who wrote:

> O blest retirement, friend of life's decline,
> Retreats from care that never must be mine,
> How happy he who crowns, in shades like these,
> A youth of labour with an age of ease;

but not necessarily blest if too much ease or too strange or distant the shades. You will, of course, pay attention to keeping fit. We should all aim to live until we die. Exercise and a modicum of restraint pay dividends.

Freedom to act

The most important aspect of retirement is activity. The individual's own inclinations and abilities will determine what activities are pursued; the best often prove to be those long thwarted by the pressures of the daily round. Retirement activities should be enjoyable. Bertrand Russell put this with his accustomed clarity in *Portraits from Memory* when he wrote: "There is need, first, of a stable framework built round a central purpose and second, of what may be called 'play', that is to say, of things that are done merely because they are fun and not because they serve some serious end."

Inner resources are the thing; with these there can be no cause for concern—activities abound. It is, however, creative activities that most certainly promote happiness, even when, as usual, they are laced with frustration. If you can paint, write music, sing in a choir, play in an orchestra, or write acceptable prose or poetry, you are fortunate indeed. I have often had to remind sceptical friends that gardening is a creative activity. Some remarkable group activities have been set up. I recently heard of one most successful theatre group and club, run exclusively by retired people, that puts on a new show each month for which it is often difficult to get a seat.

One oddity is open to you. If you harbour a qualm that your full worth may not have been appreciated, or more seriously that you have been recognised only for your less important contributions, the *British Medical Journal* encourages you to compose your own obituary. These are, of course, chiefly written for the nearest and

179

dearest at home and at work, but that need not stop you from try-ing, without too much earnestness, to avoid being one of Hardy's *Spectres that Grieve*:

> We are stript of rights; our shames lie unredressed,
> Our deeds in full anatomy are not shown,
> Our words in morsells merely are expressed
> On the scriptured page, our motives blurred unknown.

Of the essence

You must, and you will, do your own thing, but some of the suggestions I would put forward are:

(1) Take care to prepare for retirement well in advance.

(2) Arrange for continuing financial stability at whatever level is open to you. You may live a very long time.

(3) Make no too sudden break in your habit of caring for others or with your familiar surroundings.

(4) Remember that the key to happiness is activity, preferably creative.

(5) Give some thought, but not too much, to maintaining fitness and avoiding over indulgence.

(6) Have fun.

To me the essence of successful retirement was embodied in a charming, courteous gentleman, who was the ear, nose, and throat surgeon to the Brompton Hospital and the Royal Academy of Music among his many appointments. Sir James Dundas-Grant lived to be 90, and in his 80s, when I knew him as a young man, he conducted an orchestra, was straight of back, sharp of eye, and quick of thought. When asked how he managed to seem so young at his age he replied, "I say something pretty to my wife every day."

Retire: 2

GEORGE DISCOMBE

I do not know why I should be expected to give coherent advice on how to retire; rather I should receive it, because my own retirement was unplanned, was spread over 13 years, took me to Iran, to Nigeria, where I thoroughly enjoyed myself, and—when I returned after seven years' expatriation—to places as far apart as Cardiff, Basingstoke, and Inverness. Even now I am not completely retired, my present appointment being that of grandfather in attendance, in which the duties are, when required, to feed the grandchildren and their pets, occasionally to exercise them, or drive them to music lessons or to have their coats trimmed. It is quite as exacting as any of my earlier appointments, but slightly less exciting.

Strategic retreats

When you retire you give up a position of considerable authority and perforce find yourself pushed into the background. If you are an average married male your wife will have you around for most of the 24 hours of a day—and, conversely, that is longer than you really want to see her. She of course may say that she welcomes your presence, but I know of no wife who is not relieved when her husband disappears for a few hours. If you have been a working woman the results are analogous; and if you both have to retire at the same time the result may be chaos. In any case, each of you needs some refuge in which to spend much of the day. Lord Emsworth's devotion to the Empress of Blandings was a masterly subterfuge that few can attempt; clubs and societies are frequent and useful refuges, especially if one spouse displays an unyielding or tyrannical disposition (remember the triadic verb: "I am firm;

he is obstinate; you are pig headed"), but this is sometimes relieved if one party engages in non-verbal replies—though these may be interpreted as "dumb insolence" or, even worse, as complete submission.

My favourite warning was given by the—doubtless apocryphal—Quaker who was heard to say to his wife, "All the world's mad save thee and me, my dear," and then, after a short pause, "and even thee's a little bit queer." It is a salutary discipline to remember, every day before breakfast, that even if you are sure that cousin John is mad, cousin Ralph undoubtedly is sure that you are; and that if one spouse regards the other with love and admiration this does not given any assurance that the love and admiration are reciprocated. Continued courtesy and occasional exhibitions of formal respect always help; even if you still have to live with X, whose continuous sniffs, or repetition of meaningless formulas reduce you to exasperation, it is far better for you to say so, and seek a change, than to allow exasperation to break out into abuse or violence; and it is far wiser for the offender to make an effort to change, even if the complaint seems ridiculous.

By the time you are due to retire you will probably have grandchildren. All grandchildren are, in theory, heaven sent, welcome, beautiful, intelligent, and well behaved; in practice, they appear to be plain, dull, and atrociously behaved. You will be less disappointed if you assume from the time of their birth that, owing to the regression to the mean, they will fall far below your own standards of intelligence and ability; in time you will be relieved to learn that in the mother's opinion they are of somewhat above average ability, and that they do not suffer from any irrational ideas such as an excessive adoration of horses or a hatred of school. Life may then become very pleasant for all parties, the parents pleased by grandpa (ma's) obvious pleasure and the children basking in the approval of both generations—until you discover that the general opinion elsewhere is that they are spoilt little brats, an opinion endorsed by you when the parents go away and ask you to look after the little horrors.

We must cultivate our garden

All these are stages on the pilgrim's road to retirement, which indeed has some similarities to the road to Compostella, having many starting places but only one end. I think that it is more sensible to travel slowly, and that a slow retirement is wiser than a sudden stop. I was more fortunate than many, for an offer of interesting work abroad coincided with difficulties with laboratory finance at home, and so I could start the road under very favourable conditions. Nowadays it is much more difficult; Iran does not welcome foreigners, Nigeria has less money available because of the slump in oil, and many of the other organisations think that the upper age limit for consideration should be 50. It is still possible for a general practitioner to retire in phases, but much more difficult for any form of consultant, as usually the tasks he has are indivisible. For this reason private practice is desirable, but you need to have established yourself in this before you retire. The Labour party's objection to private practice, and its love of formally tidy administration, may make life very difficult for consultants who are enthusiasts, unless they are already in private practice. If you have established yourself as a writer you might retire to this with pleasure; a few individuals can find some means of continuing research, but nobody finds it easy to adapt to sudden and complete idleness.

Hobbies and clubs will become much more important in your life, but you cannot return to those of your youth. Golf, tennis, and even cricket are possible for a few years, and I find that players of outdoor games are much better tempered and harmonious than those who are physically idle. Unfortunately, many persons of retiring age are physically handicapped, and you cannot play golf when you have had attacks of recurrent sciatica or severe arthritis, either of which is likely to make you short tempered; swimming, though excellent as exercise does not occupy much of your day, and if you have gross changes produced by varicose veins you may be embarrassed at the prospect of putting them on show and possibly displeasing others. Fly fishing is getting too expensive for most people and may require absence for days rather than hours, and coarse fishing is not a pleasure for the elderly. Gardening is the common resource, and if taken moderately seriously will offer most of the benefits needed; but if there is more than one gardener in the family make sure that each one's activities are separate and well defined, for nothing is more annoying than to have some carefully tended rarity torn up because it is mistaken for a dandelion. If one wants to use "chemicals" and the other regards them with fear and loathing, you may have to separate the area tended by each. Of course you can escape much of this by employing a professional gardener, but apart from mowing the lawn and sweeping up the leaves, this takes away most of the enjoyment. Some degree of eccentric enthusiasm is here permissible, especially if you are unable to play golf or tennis; the Royal Horticultural Society, its specialist groups (I have joined the lily group and am busily trying to germinate different species), other specialist societies, and, perhaps more important, the local horticultural society, are the keys to happy gardening.

This supposes a garden, and you can rarely have a good sized garden in the middle of a city, though you can often find one in the inner suburbs. The aims of gardening in a tiny town garden are somewhat different from those in a large suburban one, but in either case moderation must be the rule—it is not sensible for a man of 65 to take on a half acre wilderness full of tree stumps unless he brings in a contractor to remove them.

Making new contacts

You may have to move to get a garden, and to move house is far more traumatic than most people suppose. If you move to another district you lose most of your friends, and even if you move locally it may be essential to establish a new circle, though this is easier in a country village than in a city; even so you might be regarded as an interloper, though this is rare nowadays. Acceptance is easier if you join some of the key societies; the first establishes your good faith—you attend the parish church if you are Church of England, and get your name on the parish roll; then join the horticultural society if you have any sort of a garden, the historical or preservation society, and, last, the political association you favour. In a city moves of much more than a mile seem to be equivalent to emigration to Australia, but suburban moves are much better tolerated. If you are moving far try to learn as much as possible of your chosen district; if an old friend lives nearby that is ideal for he/she will advise on contacts.

Of course you will enjoy entertaining at home, but there are many occasions when you or your spouse want to get out of the house and meet people who are figuratively wearing carpet slippers and sitting in their favourite armchair. This is where the village social club is so valuable; it usually contains a fair cross section of village life, professionals, craftsmen, widows, wives, and children as well as men, and will offer a great variety of relaxation; lunch or supper in mine is a minor treat for the grandchildren and useful for us all. If you join a political association you will probably get much work and meet many enthusiasts. Freemasonry offers no special advantages, though you keep contact with some old friends, but the masonic club in the nearest big town may be of some value since it sometimes offers lunch to which you may take your wife and children. It is a great disadvantage for women that they have not devised more clubs—an inevitable consequence of the division of labour in the past—though nowadays there are more in the big cities.

For some, retirement is overshadowed by some chronic and disabling illness in the spouse. The more severe forms of arthritis are slowly coming under control, but the dementias are assuming prominence—not, I think, because they are new diseases, but because more people are surviving to suffer them, and the antibiotics are, regrettably, saving the life of even advanced sufferers. The Alzheimer-like syndromes seem to be many, from one that has an onset at 55 and is fatal in five years, to another in which the sufferer has the first symptoms (very slight and indefinite) at 52, is obviously ill at 58, demented at 65, and still alive at 71. You cannot insure against these, the NHS is rarely able to take them, and you must be on the supplementary benefit level before the DHSS will do more than provide the attendance allowance, which is about £30 a week, about one quarter to one sixth of the average cost of nursing home care. This cost is tolerable if you have enough pension and some capital reserve, but if you have grandchildren who can be helped financially there will be a conflict of interest. It is essential that you have a reserve of capital at the command of either spouse, and it is quite difficult to ensure this; at some stage or another the Court of Protection may have to intervene, and its ideas are not always suitable. *Which?* recently investigated private investment advisers, and found them lacking in almost every respect; the British Medical Association should be able to give much better advice through BMA Services; but it should be possible to set up a small trust to accumulate capital in suitable unit trusts (perhaps using the new personal equity plans). A trust, set up with no more than £400 a year, using reliable unit trusts should be able to double its investments in five years, so that if this is started as soon as possible, in 10 years' time there should be enough to put the grandchildren through university, or establish them in a business, or to provide nursing.

Non-nuclear power

You will note that I am speaking, not of the nuclear family, but of a three generation family, something that has been out of favour for at least two generations. I think that one has to remember what are the great advantages of three generations—greater financial security for all, greater security in social terms, and, if there is only one grandparent, the fact that usually he/she can be fitted into the existing establishment. But most important is the recognition of the extended family, meaning all members of the earliest generation living, and all their descendants; it is surprising how much each can help the others—and always indirectly. In the area which speaks some Iranian language—Iran, Pakistan, Afghanistan, and parts of India—and in subSaharan Africa, this has always been remembered, and indeed, we lost it only during the nineteenth century when it was essential to eliminate nepotism from the law and from the civil service. It remains in these other countries, where it is of great advantage for the individual, but of doubtful value to the country as a whole; can we recover the advantages while excluding the evils?

For a wifeless man in his later 70s my family provides better care than any protected housing with a warden. I lead a reasonably active life, and in September with my sister drove through France to the Auvergne and on to Provence and back; she comes here for Glyndebourne, and I have just returned from a fortnight with her in Dorset, where we also visited a couple of cousins. At home I have cleared away three self sown cherries about 12 ft tall, several old stumps, and am now removing a very large sycamore root. Yesterday I completed a nursery bed about 18 by 4 ft and counted my perennials for next year—they include 30 each of pansies, primroses, and polyanthus, and nearly as many penstemon, kniphofia and hollyhock. There were at the last count 96 lilies, and four pots of lilies which show delayed germination and are now being chilled. As the other members of the family were busy I did most of the domestic ironing, and started to prepare for a cassoulet using turkey drumsticks instead of goose. Today or tomorrow I shall go to the nursing home to see my wife. Next week comes my 78th birthday.

Get a letter in the newspapers

CHARLES PITHER

Giles felt *so* incensed about it that he wrote to the paper . . .

Giles, rather than chaining himself to the railings, lobbying his member of parliament, or hijacking a jumbo jet, has found the ultimate vent for his spleen.

Whether it is just another nuance of Englishness like crumpets or cricket, or maybe the hope of restoring the misplaced balance of justice, or perhaps the egotistical motivation of seeing your name in print is uncertain. What is clearer is that ever since there have been newspapers "Incensed of Ipswich" and "Angry of Angmering" have been bashing off letters whenever the mood takes them. For the average man in the street there exists, beyond high dudgeon and extreme annoyance, somewhere between shaking with rage and blinding fury, a state of indignation and agitation adequately extinguished only by picking up a pen and writing to the press.

For most of us this compulsion to share our angst with the readership of a national newspaper is only an occasional phenomenon, motivated by a particular event which we feel that we cannot let pass without comment. There are, however, a group of gallant scribes in perpetual competition with themselves, who dispatch letters with the same regularity as they consume their All Bran. For them the game is simply to get into print at any cost, and, although volume of letters is one approach, it is by no means guaranteed to succeed.

Whether a letter published in a national newspaper ever makes any difference to the subject is questionable. At best it certainly may bring a point to the notice of a wide readership, at worst the author can feel that at least he did something about the injustice nagging at his conscience. The more pertinent consideration, however, is how to get the editor to publish it in the first place. Having made the decision that sleep will be impossible until the ancient typewriter has been dusted off and loaded with crisp foolscap, what are the mysterious ingredients that secure publication?

There is a tendency to believe that most of the successful authors are dons, lords, members of the Athenaeum, chairmen of royal commissions, or country curates, but the evidence disputes this. Although there are, not surprisingly, a large number of letters from eminent persons of all walks of life, the majority of letters published come from untitled, ordinary people who never have, nor ever will, be regius professor of Egyptian archaeology at Oxford. A large number of letters do appear from doctors, but it is pertinent to remember PhD, DPhil, DD, etc, as they frequently enable you to dissociate yourself from a viewpoint totally inexplicable had it come from within the medical profession.

The choice of subject is, of course, dependent upon the motivation of the instant, and I can give little advice about this. The small earthquake in Ongar may, you feel, have deserved greater treatment, or Goethe's original meaning have been misconstrued in a new translation. Your comment may be topical or pertinent enough to merit publication on this alone, but there are several factors that can be helpful.

Headed notepaper is certainly worth while especially if the letter is on the serious side. The editor himself won't know much about forensic psychiatry and so if your comment appears on paper headed "Academic Department of Forensic Psychiatry" it may carry more weight. The same applies to qualifications; put them all in and hope to blind them with science. Likewise it is worth considering joint signatories, which is a good idea if they add weight to your case. Although the length of the letter in itself is not critical, you are unlikely to repeat Jefferies's 1862 success with his missive of 3000 words on the plight of agricultural labourers. It is more important to be succinct and to the point, conveying, as in a scientific paper, your exact meaning with the minimum of superfluous words.

Lines of approach

When it comes to style, it is worth remembering that there are several styles of letter that appear time and time again, the use of which may modify, for better or worse, the letter's chance of actually appearing in print.

The Tunbridge Wells

This is the letter which from the first line conjures up the image of a bristling moustache upon the quivering upper lip of a retired general. The *Daily Telegraph* letters page consists almost entirely of letters such as this. The subjects range widely from the union jack being upside down on Remembrance Sunday (. . . what's the country coming to, etc, etc) to the union jack being upside down on Boxing Day (. . . what has the country come to, etc). In general not a recommended approach especially to the more liberal organs.

The Bernard Shaw

In spite of these observations, if you do happen to be a revered household name of advancing years, it is going to be a very stalwart editor who would deny you column inches in his paper. If you have not been heard from for the past 10 years so much the better. The content of your letter is unimportant but it may as well be on something totally trivial. This will give the nation the pleasure of confirmation that you really are senile and, as they suspected, quietly dementing.

The trireme

This is perhaps the best approach for the enthusiastic amateur. Success depends upon two things. Firstly, knowing a great amount about an aspect of a subject so minimal that most of the population did not know there even was a subject, and, secondly, a lead or introduction. This is the problem; while it is not too difficult to become an expert in a specialised topic it is all too easy to die waiting for an opportunity to tell the world all about it. The best solution to this problem is obliquity:

Sir,
Your article on the closure of the Tuileries gallery made no mention of the famous carp to be found in the ornamental ponds of the *jardin*. These fish and others of the family are particularly prone to a fungus *Hyspericillus inpratroides* that over a period of time damages the ventral fin and thus causes the fish to swim

around in circles. While this is not detrimental in the round ponds of Paris the situation in the natural habitat in Xi'ang province etc, etc.

If you are very lucky, somewhere in the depths of a crumbling university a don of great learning, total obscurity, and an age best ascertained by carbon dating, will disagree and will write to the editor saying so. If all goes well the whole nation can then delight in the joys of a correspondence to which most of its premier minds contribute, in thought if not in publication.

The anti

The majority of the letters in all the serious papers. The best way the editor has of appeasing his conscience if he has published libel, controversy, or fiction. The letter simply states with convincing evidence that the article or implication was misguided/wrong/ libellous/damned lies. The problem is that in these circumstances the mail bag will be full of similar letters and yours must be outstanding to get in with a chance. This can be achieved by taking a totally contrary view, or by being a member of the Athenaeum, chairman of a royal commission, etc.

The bottom right hand corner

The traditional position in *The Times* where letters of some wit, originality, or total irrelevance end up. The best chance of publication is to find something of such amusing eccentricity or idiocy that the editor has no option but to publish. If this something happens to be yourself, publication is almost guaranteed.

Luck and judgment

This is, of course an attempt at categorising a subject not very amenable to such treatment. Probably the best way of getting your letter into print is to avoid all these approaches and come up with something completely original and imaginatively different.

Having written the letter, crammed with pertinent comment, brilliant innovation, cutting wit, and a deal of eccentricity, you read it through 10 times, tear it up, and start again. Eventually you end up with a compromise with which you are least unhappy, and rush to the post office to catch the last post. Then you have the awful waiting. Although there is no chance of publication the following morning, you buy the paper and scan the letters page just on the off chance that the editor sent a courier round to your letter box specially. The next few days you spring to the newsagent and scan the letters page even before the cost of the paper has changed hands. Usually it is a progressive disappointment. After a week all thoughts of the editor "saving it for the weekend because it's so good" can be dismissed and the only consolation will be the nice letter from the editor's assistant saying that the editor read your comments with interest. If, of course, yours was one of the 300 letters received that day to be published, the problem is then whether by going out to lunch to celebrate you might miss the call from *Panorama* requesting your appearance on a studio panel. Either way you will dine out on it for weeks, perhaps months, or— for some old bores—the rest of your life.

If you are unlucky and the Wapping rejection slip drops on to the door mat, nothing matters less. In seismological terms the earthquake in Ongar was a non-starter, and maybe the new translation of Goethe is actually better. The therapeutic effect of writing to a newspaper is in the writing not in the publication. In fact on odd occasions the letter may not even get as far as the letter box. One of the best letters ever received by *The Times* was from a Major Wintle:

Sir,
I have just written you a long letter.
   On reading it through I have thrown it into the waste paper basket.
   Hoping this meets with your approval,
     I am, Sir,
   Your obedient servant,

Giles, like Major Wintle, will still feel greatly relieved that he did actually write, and he will inform his friends regardless of whether his letter was published or not. Writing to newspapers is an integral part of being a concerned citizen, and, as doctors, we frequently have reason to be concerned. This is a particularly British way of doing things. No other race could have masterminded an effective form of protest that does not even entail getting out of a chair.

In the words of René Gimpel, an Englishman is "A man with a passion for horses, playing with a ball, probably one broken bone in his body and in his pocket a letter to *The Times*."

Long may it continue.

Write an obituary

A G W WHITFIELD

What is the purpose of an obituary? Certainly not to notify death, for bad news travels fast and patients, colleagues, and friends will usually hear of a doctor's decease within hours rather than days. Its main objective, like the address at the funeral, is to give solace to the bereaved family. To read their loved one's achievements and good qualities extolled in carefully chosen words of eulogy undoubtedly gives comfort and a feeling of pride which to some extent mitigates grief. A kind and good obituary evokes gratitude from those who mourn while one which underestimates its subject is swiftly met with resentment and anger, and nothing can "wash out a word of it."

An important secondary objective is of maintaining esprit de corps. If when a St Monica's man dies his colleagues all attend his memorial service, one giving an oration thereat, while another writes a generous tribute for *The Times* or *British Medical Journal*, it all helps to maintain the prestige of St Monica's, and this applies in the same way to the medical community of a county town, the medical service of the navy, army, or air force or any other medical body. A third function of the obituary is to provide posterity with a fragment of accurate medical history of the period. The purpose of an obituary is certainly not to try to convince the world of the greatness of the man who has died, whose existence was unknown to all but a few when he was alive.

The length of an obituary will largely be decided by the journal for which it is being written and to which it must be exclusively submitted. Unless your subject was someone of very great national importance half a dozen double column inches is the maximum that *The Times* will be able to print and if a cabinet minister or film star happens to choose the same day on which to die even this may be curtailed. On the other hand an obituary written for inclusion in

Biographical Memoirs of Fellows of the Royal Society may stretch to any length the writer has the strength to produce. Medical journals, particularly the *British Medical Journal* and the *Lancet*, are under great pressure for space and the editor of the *British Medical Journal* now asks for contributions to be restricted to about 400 words. Naturally this allows little scope for non-essentials.

Speak of me as I am

What therefore should an obituary include and exclude? While none of us of course knows, it seems unlikely that in the next world we shall have to apply and compete for consultant vacancies. In fact, in that undiscovered country it may be that we shall be allotted humble and distasteful work to equalise for the privileged position, the high salary, and the index linked pension that we have enjoyed here. Obituaries should not therefore consist of a curriculum vitae with a list of qualifications and experience that could be used for job applications on the other side of the river. In fact the obituary's content should be confined to what is interesting and important and it should endeavour to paint a portrait and capture the spirit of the man. De mortuis nil nisi bonum should be carved deep on the author's desk, but no man is without blemish and no life is free from fault. To omit the weaker facets and to stress the good qualities is essential but the canvas must also show the special attributes and skills, the humour or lack of it, the leisure interests, and the many different attitudes and beliefs which together made up the man whose life we are striving to honour in generous perspective. Strict factual accuracy is essential. No children reach for their pen more quickly than those whose father is erroneously recorded as having been president when he was in fact the assistant secretary. In the *Journal of the American Medical Association* the cause of death is usually included, but thankfully not on this side of the Atlantic. It cannot give pleasure to relatives to read that death was due to alcoholic cirrhosis of the liver or syphilitic aortitis. In any case inaccurate death certification seems to be almost as certain as death.

Gathering detail for an obituary may prove difficult. *Who's Who*, the *Medical Directory*, the *Medical Register* and college lists provide a good deal of information but it is usually necessary to approach a member of the family about some items and it is a revelation to find how often they are unable to help in filling the gap.

You should include a photograph if you can obtain one which is neither too out of date nor too uncomplimentary. The family, hospital, or medical school or a friend will usually be able to find one that they are willing to lend but if not the portrait libraries hold an enormous number and can often help.

The family of the deceased should be mentioned, particularly if any of them have entered the medical profession, but however distinguished they may have become it is important to do little more than mention them—it is not their obituary that you are writing.

The opening paragraph should state, "John Henry Smith, the well known physician from Much Binding in the Marsh, died in hospital on 1 April" and then the date and place of birth, parentage, and short particulars of scholastic, university, and postgraduate education should follow. Two or three lines is all that is required for this unless there are some features that would be of especial interest to readers.

Many hospitals and medical schools, realising the importance of good obituaries, insist on anyone appointed to their staff completing a proforma of biographical details and updating it every five years. In addition, many designate a senior member of staff to be responsible for writing, or persuading a suitable colleague to write, an appropriate tribute when the time arrives. Although such co-ordinators are sometimes said to add another terror to death, if some arrangement of this nature is not made hurtful omissions are inevitable. If it is left to the subeditor of a journal to invite an obituary his request may reach someone who did not hold his deceased colleague in high regard, with embarrassing results. Certainly you should decline a request to contribute an obituary of someone for whom you had feelings of contempt or dislike, and an editor or subeditor might perhaps most suitably approach the dean of the medical school or the appropriate professor when seeking an obituarist. For general practitioners the British Medical Association will have little difficulty in suggesting the most suitable person. The best obituaries, however, tend to come from those who have been colleagues and personal friends of the subject, and his family will often express this preference or make their own approach.

Advance notices

Many editors keep obituaries ready for publication for figures of great eminence or advanced age or who are known to be mortally ill so that they may be promptly published. This is not only good journalism but it is a very acceptable compliment to the deceased. In fact an obituary loses a proportion of its value with every day that passes between death and publication. An additional advantage is that it allows the editor time to consider who would be the most fitting person from whom to request the tribute. The undesirability of delay is reflected by the rule of the editor of the *British Medical Journal* not to publish an obituary more than six months after a person's death.

"Write your own" is just beginning and it has the advantage that obituaries so compiled are likely to be factually correct and that they will be ready for publication as soon as death occurs. It is as yet too early to know to what extent this practice will prove acceptable and become current coin. The obvious difficulty will be of the modest and self effacing undervaluing their worth and the egoistic and self satisfied painting too flattering a portrait of themselves.

There are many volumes of biography made up of obituaries of varying quality. The standard of those in the *Dictionary of National Biography*, *Munk's Roll*, *Plarr's Lives*, *The Times*, the *British Medical Journal* and the *Lancet* is high but writing an obituary is, like any literary skill, an art that requires time and practice to acquire, and some never succeed. An obituary is as much a measure of the writer and his relationship with the subject as it is of the subject himself and many are so apt and moving as to become part of our nation's heritage. Dr Samuel Johnson's obituary poem to Robert Levett, whom he had known for over 40 years, was a wonderful example of how to write an obituary, and his tribute to his lifelong friend, David Garrick, whose death "eclipsed the gaiety of nations and impoverished the public stock of harmless pleasure," will live forever.

Write for money

MICHAEL O'DONNELL

Don't tell the editor, or at least not till after I've been paid, but I am not a good person to give advice about writing for money. I'm unusually lucky in that I've survived by writing what I want to write and then finding someone willing to publish it. It is not a course I'd recommend to anyone concerned with making money. I could call my bank manager as witness.

The nearest I get to a direct bid for the lucre is when I accept a commission for an article, or a script, on a subject I haven't chosen for myself and try to deliver what I hope is expected. But even then the most valuable reward is not the payment—though it can produce a comfortable feeling in the pocket—but the discipline that the exercise imposes. (Again I beg you, gentle reader, please don't tell the editor until he's signed the cheque.)

Publish and be educated

Like everyone else, I find writing a laborious business and I'm sure that if my working habits came under the scrutiny of one of those city analysts who have proliferated under our present regime with the exuberance of thistles in a cow byre, he would consult his Filofax and say I spend too much time writing things that offer a low financial return per mmol of sweated blood. He would, I'm sure, advise me to desist from writing novels and return to writing the television plays I wrote when I was harder up, or advertisements for Snibbo or for Treadgold's Thoroughgrip Garterettes. Just as he would demand that I should never again write for such ill paying publications as ... but this is no place to be naming names. The problem with Filofax man, of course, is that while he is good at measuring returns he has no measure of rewards.

That said, let us consider this business of earning money.

Doctor writers if they can make any show of competence should find it easier than other writers to get their work published. Thanks to the money spent on pharmaceutical promotion, medical publications have proliferated almost as exuberantly as city analysts. One or two are first rate but the content of some reveals the strain their editors are under to find something to keep the advertisements apart. These are useful places for medical writers to learn their craft. Nearly all the cliches uttered about writing are true, so I don't apologise for repeating the truism that the only way to learn how to write is to write, and to keep on writing. This dreary business of churning out words can be lightened by occasional publication, and doctors are lucky to have a group of editors who are more likely to read their work, comment on it, and even publish it, than the hard faced persons who sit in editors' chairs elsewhere.

Doctors also have an advantage when submitting their work to non-medical magazines and newspapers. People, not surprisingly, are interested in their health. More surprisingly, they are also interested in the antics of doctors. So practising doctors who write about their work simply, directly, and with enthusiasm, have a good chance of selling "A doctor writes . . ." style articles. The late Dr Alfred Byrne, a hardened Fleet Street correspondent, used to call it "working the bronchitis belt."

Easy reading, hard writing

The key words in that last paragraph are "enthusiasm," "simply," and "directly." If, when you write an article, you can generate no enthusiasm for its subject—a state into which it is easy to lapse if you concentrate only on the lucre—it will quickly bore any reader foolish enough to dip into it, no matter how much technical skill you deploy on its construction. Similarly, unless you can express what you want to say in simple direct prose, much of what you write will remain unread.

It is not easy to be simple and direct. One writing doctor, W Somerset Maugham, claimed: "To write simply is as difficult as to be good." If anything, he understated the problem. Yet achieving an appearance of simplicity is the central skill of the writer's craft. Luckily help is at hand, set out in useful textbooks. My favourite is *The Elements of Style* by Strunk and White,[1] a slim volume which contains everything we need to know but will never master in our lifetimes. For more specialised help, I recommend *Thorne's Better Medical Writing*.[2]

These books describe the simple techniques which underpin our craft. The techniques are easy to understand; the problems—and the hard work—come when we try to apply them. It is dangerous to be dogmatic about writing but here cometh a dogmatic statement that is as near as dammit true. To forge simple direct prose you need to rewrite and rewrite and rewrite and rewrite. An article such as this, for instance, needs to be rewritten at least 20 times. But once again help is at hand in the shape of that electronic marvel called a word processor.

Mechanical and moral support

Any writers who still use typewriters or who, as I once did, use pen and paper, are burdening themselves with unnecessary manual work which is not only tedious but wholly unproductive. The only drawback to using a word processor is that we no longer know how many times we rewrite, and that is a drawback only to the boastful. Gone are those piles of paper, smothered with crossings out and arrows, waiting for a competent typist to produce the final "clean copy" which, of course, never was the final copy and had to be retyped again and again as the words sank beneath the inky tide of corrections.

Thanks to the word processor, writing and rewriting are welded into a seamless process and even a stumbling typist like me can produce printed words which, if naught else, are at least legible. God help us but it's true that some publishers and editors still make their first judgment of the quality of a manuscript on the neatness of its presentation. So if you get your magic machine to type your words double spaced on A4 paper, you're off to a flying start.

That's when you'll need another class of textbook. The best guide to where the money lies is the *Writers' and Artists' Year Book*[3] which lists all the people likely to buy your wares, tells you what they are after, and hints at what they are likely to pay. When it comes to protecting yourself in this jungle, the medical profession is, once again, twice blessed. Two patient support groups exist to help innocent doctors who stray into the threatening world of editors and publishers: the Medical Writers' Group within the Society of Authors (84 Drayton Gardens, London SW10 9SB), and the GP Writers' Association, which can be contacted through Dr David Haslam, 33 Biggin Lane, Huntingdon, Cambridgeshire.

When contracts grow complicated, as they can with books and television programmes, it's well worth acquiring an agent. A brazen agent will get you more money from publishers than you'd dare ask for yourself—usually more than the 10% which is the only commission a reputable agent will demand. The *Writers' and Artists' Year Book* includes a list of agents and advice on how to approach them.

Yet no matter how brazen your agent, only you can earn the money. So it's back to simplicity, directness, and a word processor, which when deployed with enthusiasm, may warm the cockles of your bank manager's heart and allow you to eat occasional slices of cake instead of bread. If, however, you are tempted to try to make writing your main occupation rather than a part time one, you will need to make more drastic changes to your way of life. Once you start writing for a living, you cannot rely only on technique. You need to cultivate a way of living that feeds your imagination, and you need to discover more about the creature who produces the words, the voice that speaks to the reader when you write. This demands some dedicated introspection because, unless you write with some honesty of purpose, and try honestly to express the complexities within you and which you see around you, your writing will smack of triteness.

To write from any motive other than honesty is to write propaganda. That may not deter you if your only aim is to make money. Propaganda is certainly a profitable form of writing. It demands the same skills and techniques as any other writing and suits many people as a well paid part time occupation. It is, however, thin gruel to sustain the enthusiasm of a full time writer (am I using enthusiasm as a euphemism for obsession?) and you can measure its charm by reading political pamphlets or watching party political broadcasts.

Profit of penitence

I have left the most practical advice till last because it is also the most painful. I have yet to meet anybody who finds the business of setting down words a pleasurable way of passing the time. All of us who write yearn for diversions that will take us away from the desk or from the keyboard or, even better, some urgent matter that will prevent us from even starting. Most writers of my acquaintance compel themselves to write a certain number of words, or to spend a specified time at their desk, every day. Some of the best prose they produce may come during a session which got off to a reluctant start; some sessions which grow out of bubbling enthusiasm may produce only rubbish.

The secret of successful writing is, as Mother Mary Catherine hinted all those years ago on my very first day at school, a matter of self discipline, and the appropriate working garb is sackcloth and ashes. Still, it seems to do no great harm to most of us to play the penitent for a few hours every day—and it does bring temporal rewards. The greater the suffering while the stuff's being hammered out, the greater the joy when we reach the last full stop.

Forgive that late intrusion by Samuel Smiles (another doctor writer, as it happens), but I can sense the final marker racing towards me. The cheque, I trust, will soon be in the post.

1   Strunk W, White E B. *The elements of style*. New York: Macmillan, 1972.
2   Lock S. *Thorne's better medical writing*. London: Pitman, 1977.
3   *The writers' and artists' yearbook*. London: A and C Black.

Choose a better word

B J FREEDMAN

In nineteenth century England all doctors learnt Latin at school and some learnt Greek too. In that epoch the use of long words, derived from Greek and Latin roots, was regarded as the mark of good style. I believe this to have been the natural enjoyment derived from using an acquired skill. It served, incidentally, to render the language more intelligible internationally. Latin and Greek have virtually fallen by the wayside, and in their stead English is fast becoming, or has perhaps already become, the international language of medicine. The trend, therefore, is to return to its Anglo-Saxon roots. This is resulting in shorter, and often clearer, words. At the same time there is a trend to simplify syntax and to express one's thoughts more clearly. There is, however, a steady trickle of polysyllabic latinised neologisms embedded in convoluted clauses, which emanates from a few, mainly American, writers. I suspect that these aspects of style derive from the Italian and German components of the linguistic melting pot.

Lists of words and phrases for which more suitable alternatives are recommended have been compiled by Bill Whimster,[1] Stephen Lock,[2] and Raymond Whitehead[3] and are well worth reading. My purpose here is to mention some of my bêtes noires, to say why I think they are better avoided, and to suggest alternatives.

Fashionable jargon

OVERWEIGHT was introduced, I think, to avoid giving offence to the well educated who were obese, and to the plebs who were too fat. Through frequent use it has unfortunately established itself in clinical terminology; unfortunately, because it is sometimes diagnosed merely by reference to tables of average or ideal body weight, and without always taking the simple precaution of looking at the unclothed patient. Some people who are overweight by this definition are stocky, muscular, and lean, yet they may be wrongly labelled overweight in the sense of obese. We are currently in a permissive age of vernacular speech. So why not say, "Madam, you are too fat?"

COMPARABLE. Two things are comparable if they can be set together so as to ascertain to what extent they agree or disagree.

If two formulations have comparable bioavailability then we can expect them to have the same clinical effect.

"Similar" is the right word.

Vogue words

SPIRAL and ESCALATION are vogue words for "increase," especially in a pejorative sense.

The question of whether the BBC . . . is the best way to preserve public service broadcasting against the pressures of spiralling costs . . . remains unanswered.

A spiral may be flat like a volute or the balance spring of a watch, or it may be a helix like a spiral staircase. It is this latter image, with a vertical axis, that is intended. It may be more than coincidental that the metaphorical use of spiral seems to have begun after the dramatic publicisation of the DNA double helix. When so specified, spirals can also go down.

The dangers of the descending spiral to law enforcement . . . have been repeated for many years.

ESCALATION is geometrically more appropriate and will probably stay.

Medical negligence claims have escalated rapidly since the beginning of the last decade.

When is a synonym not a synonym?

TREATMENT and THERAPY are synonymous terms. THERAPY is sometimes more suited to a literary style, and it is the rule in combining forms, as in "radiotherapy." The advocates of "fringe" treatments prefer to call their methods alternative therapies, presumably because the magniloquence of THERAPY is thought to invest the discipline with a greater sense of importance than would TREATMENT. I have no quarrel with this—well, not much—but when the word THERAPY is used without qualification to mean "alternative therapy," then the word becomes debased. I quote:

VAT ... is a tax on the freedom of choice for medical attention on those patients who prefer to have therapeutic treatment. (House of Lords.)

MANUAL versus HANDBOOK. The reviewer of a book wrote:

Truly a manual rather than a handbook, it should be recommended to trainees in rheumatology and orthopaedics.

A handbook is a manual (Latin *manus*, hand).

The postmortem examination

NECROPSY, AUTOPSY, and BIOPSY. Necropsy and autopsy are synonyms. Though AUTOPSY is slighly easier in speech, it is etymologically less satisfactory since the derivation implies "seeing for oneself" (corpse understood). By derivation NECROPSY specifies that a corpse is under examination. One word is enough, and NECROPSY is to be preferred. I thought everyone knew that BIOPSY meant examining a piece of tissue removed from a living subject until I read:

Full postmortem examination was not carried out but percutaneous biopsy specimens of liver and spleen showed ...

Pitfalls exist when communicating with Greeks, for whom *necropsia* means external examination of a corpse, while our necropsy is their *necrotomē*. Worse still, their *autopsia* means any sort of specialist inspection, for example, of the scene of a crime or earthquake damage.[4]

When we don't know the cause

PRIMARY, ESSENTIAL, IDIOPATHIC, SPONTANEOUS, and CRYPTO-GENIC are epithets used for conditions whose cause is unknown. The first three went into a decline after the last war, but have regained their popularity in recent years.

PRIMARY is used in contradistinction to "secondary." In the 1930s secondary anaemias were those due to bleeding or malnutrition; the primary anaemias were those with no apparent cause, such as pernicious anaemia. For obvious reasons that epithet for anaemia has been dropped, but PRIMARY is very much with us, and I have seen it currently applied to immunodeficiency disease, glaucoma, Raynaud's phenomenon, erythromelalgia, pruritus ani, and lymphoedema. It should be unnecessary to say that we are not here concerned with PRIMARY in the context of tumours.

ESSENTIAL does not mean one must try to get it regardless of cost. A good definition in the medical context is that in the *Oxford English Dictionary* (marked "obsolete"): "dependent on the intrinsic character or condition of anything—not on extraneous circumstances." It has been applied to arterial hypertension and to thrombocytopenic purpura for many years and to these it must now be regarded as fixed, but recent accretions are benign haematuria and thrombocythaemia.

IDIOPATHIC. The Greek root *idio-* means own, personal, private. In a medical context, therefore, IDIOPATHIC was applied to conditions that were not related to anything else. IDIOPATHIC has been applied to epilepsy for many decades, but it has recently burgeoned into Parkinson's disease, ulceration of the small bowel, mediastinal fibrosis, neurogenic anorectal incontinence, scoliosis, "severe anaemia," hyperhidrosis, tinnitus, deafness, persistent hepatitis, and disseminated skeletal hyperostosis.

SPONTANEOUS, as applied, for example, to pneumothorax, likewise implies an origin de novo and without apparent cause.

Every condition has its cause. When we don't know the cause, what better term is there then CRYPTOGENIC (Gk *kryptos*, hidden + *genesis*, origin)—in the absence of a single Anglo-Saxon derivation? CRYPTOGENIC is the currently used epithet for certain forms of fibrosing alveolitis, cirrhosis, and chronic persistent hepatitis. Whether or not CRYPTOGENIC is found acceptable, it is manifestly absurd to have a random choice of five terms for the same thing. If we abandoned the terms PRIMARY, ESSENTIAL, IDIOPATHIC, and SPONTANEOUS, which are incompatible with twentieth century thinking, in favour of CRYPTOGENIC it would clarify and unify the terminology of the unknown.

Wrong usage

HEALTHY for WHOLESOME, as in the following quotations.

Fish is healthy food.

Most Germans believe that natural foods are better and more healthy than artificial foods.

Food is not HEALTHY; it may be WHOLESOME and those who eat

WHOLESOME food are more likely to be HEALTHY than those who do not. The German *gesund* has both meanings, and the misuse in English may be an importation.

METHODOLOGY for METHOD. METHODOLOGY is the study of methods, for example, a comparison of different methods of evaluating the same drug. It should not be used when METHOD is the right word.

> The methodology of all three papers had much in common.

This would have been better written as "The three papers described similar methods."

DISINTEREST for LACK OF INTEREST, and DISINTERESTED for UN-INTERESTED.

> The specialist journals are being filled with papers written out of necessity and read with disinterest.

The writer meant "without interest." DISINTERESTED means unbiased by personal interest, impartial.

BEG for ASK (or PUT) THE QUESTION.

> That begs the interesting question—what is the minimum workload for a surgeon (or indeed a physician) if he or she is to maintain competence?

> The first question begs another: what is pulmonary surfactant?

To beg the question is to assume what is to be proved as part of the proof. It is an error in logical thinking. It does not mean "ask the question" or "beg leave to put the question."

Wrong spelling

There is little to be said here. I believe that bad spellers are born, and that nothing much can be done to help this minority. For the average speller the remedy is to have a handy sized dictionary within easy reach. This means, for the occupants of houses, having one upstairs and one downstairs. I recommend *Chambers 20th Century Dictionary*. Learning Latin at school helps, but it is not worth while taking it up in later life merely to improve your English.

When writing for publication, you have a subeditor to correct spelling errors (and straighten out the syntax). There are, however, two words that commonly slip through the editorial net. WEAL, not "wheal." WEAL is from Old English and meant originally a ridge, hence now a raised ridge or spot on the skin. The word became confused with "wheal," also Old English, meaning a pustule. HYPERCAPNIA and its cousin "hypocapnia," not "hypercapnoea." This error has arisen from a mistaken belief that -pnia has something to do with breathing and should be spelt -pnoea. The relevant root is Gk *kapnos*, smoke. In this context smoke stands for carbon dioxide, whence hyper/capnia means too much CO_2 in the blood, or in modern terms, a raised blood CO_2 tension.

WHO and WHOM. Confusion between these two is not a question of spelling, but may conveniently be dealt with here. The tabloid newspapers seem to go out of their way to consolidate the confusion. I quote (not from a tabloid):

It is now policy to start nasogastric feeding in patients whom we think will be ventilated for a long time.

Omit "we think" and it is obvious that it is "patients WHO will be ventilated."

Ambiguities

CONTEMPORARY used as an adjective, means belonging to the same time, age, or period. The same time as what? And when? The context usually gives the answer—but not always; and that is where ambiguity may arise.

Most of these defects arose from the limited experimental information available to Carnot at the time and the imperfect state of contemporary knowledge.

... premiered in 1877, it links music and speech in a ... way that won the composer great contemporary acclaim.

CONTEMPORARY in the above obviously refers to time past.

Contemporary issues in clinical immunology.
Contemporary gastroenteritis in infants.

In these two examples CONTEMPORARY just as obviously refers to the present. It is where the text deals with times both past and present that there is risk of ambiguity, for example:

The characters of Sneer and Mr Dangle are warped prototypes ... with more pretensions but less power than their contemporary equivalents.

The foundation of Johns Hopkins Medical School in 1889 ... led to a scientific revolution ... illustrated by 51 ... articles originally published in the journal together with a contemporary comment by an expert.

I suggest that, where there is a possibility of ambiguity, and the context permits, "modern" or "present day" be substituted. CONTEMPORARY is pushing "modern" into obsolescence. Revive the use of "modern," say I.

UNCOOPERATIVE can mean "unable to" or "unwilling to," and unless the distinction is made clear, serious misunderstanding can occur. This is more likely to arise in case notes than in manuscripts for publication.

COMPROMISE. To COMPROMISE, in a clinical context, is to put at risk, to jeopardise. Correctly used in:

Many of these functions are compromised . . . in the healthy aged.

COMPROMISED has drifted semantically to mean also impaired.

. . . and when this exceeds the normal capillary blood pressure the arterial supply to the muscles is compromised.

Here "impaired" would be better, or more specifically "blocked." Because present usage of COMPROMISE may mean either "impair" or "jeopardise" (put at risk of impairment), it is preferable to say which one means.

Laymen's language

When speaking to patients, use words to which they are accustomed. It is debatable, however, whether the vernacular style is suited to medical writing. I quote:

. . . vaginal bleeding with an ectopic pregnancy can be mistaken for a period.

Care is needed where the vernacular adopts quasimedical terms. I overheard a colleague inquire about a patient's way of life. He said, "And what is your biggest headache?" In the context of his questioning this was obviously a metaphorical headache, but one which could be taken literally by a simple soul or by a foreigner.

Metaphors

Metaphors are better avoided in scientific writing, even though their occasional use may enliven an otherwise dull discussion. By their unintelligibility they may baffle those readers whose first language is not English, and who are unacquainted with our allusive phrases. For example, it may mean nothing to a foreign reader to be told that a particular sign is the HALLMARK of a certain condition, when we wish to imply that it is pathognomonic. Recourse to a dictionary, only to discover that it means *contrôle* or *Feingehaltsstempel*, will add to the confusion.

Needless syllables

In the opening paragraph I mentioned the entry into medical writing of polysyllabic neologisms and the counter current towards short Saxon rooted words, and I implied a strong preference for the latter on the grounds of clarity and better understanding. Unfortunately, once a long word is established it is not readily shortened. Nevertheless, in the past two decades we have seen "valvular" and "valvulotomy" shorted to VALVAR and VALVOTOMY, and heart sounds that were once reduplicated are now DUPLICATED. Good for the cardiologists. Practitioners in other specialties please note.

I conclude by offering for thought a few suggestions for change in this direction. I do not, however, expect miracles.

Readers will not be surprised to hear that the General Medical Services Committee has reiterated its opposition to the government's plan.

To ITERATE is to repeat or perform a second time; to "reiterate" is to do so a third time or more.

People will continue to MICTURATE in future as they have done in the past, yet I would not be the first to point out that the root of "micturate" and "micturition" is the Latin *micturio*, to desire to urinate. The Latin for urinate is *mingo*, past participle *mictum*. This would give us MINGATE for the action and MICTION for the process. How strange that in speech the sixteenth letter of the alphabet suffices.

1 Whimster W F. Be your own subeditor. *How to do it*. Vol 1. 2nd edn. London: British Medical Journal, 1987: 220–3.
2 Lock S. *Thorne's better medical writing*. 2nd edn. Tunbridge Wells: Pitman Medical, 1977.
3 Whitehead R. English for doctors. *Lancet* 1956; ii: 390–3.
4 Dafforn-Ierodiakonou E. Necrotomy, necropsy, and autopsy. *Br Med J* 1983; 287: 840.

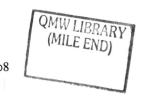